C000263682

ISBN: 9798652166816

Independently published

Copyright Tamara Cianfini 2020

This work was produced in collaboration with Write Business Results Ltd.

For more information on Write Business Results' author services,

please visit our website or feel free to contact us:

www.writebusinessresults.com

020 3752 7057

info@writebusinessresults.com

Important message for all choosing to attend a hypnobirthing course:

Hypnobirthing is NOT an alternative to medical advice. Should you have any concerns at any point during your pregnancy please consult with your medical care providers.

Contents

Contents

Path 3: The B.R.E.A.T.H. Path

Path 4: The B.A.B.Y. Path

Dedication

There is no single dedication in this book because each path travelled intertwines with the next and each carries equal importance. Crossing paths with the following people has inspired me to create this modern hypnobirthing book for you and your birth partner.

- Frankie, my son, and the vital lessons learnt throughout his traumatic birth.

- My doula Suzanne Howlett who showed me the way and totally believed in me.

- Marie Mongan, an inspirational pioneer of hypnobirthing.

- Sandy Riley, my amazing mum who supported me throughout both births.

- Alana, my daughter, whose birth totally opened my eyes to new and unimaginable possibilities that led me down a new and exciting path as a hypnobirthing teacher.

I didn't write this book alone. It is a product of all the passionate hypnobirthing teachers and parents who have crossed my path since I discovered it in 2007. I have weaved the wisdom and passion that they have shared with me throughout this book.

Preface:

The Birth Path

It is in the journey that the way becomes more clear! *The Birth Path* will show you the way to achieve a successful hypnobirth for you and your baby. The knowledge and wisdom weaved throughout each of the four paths before reaching 'The Birth Path' will help you feel more prepared and ready to meet your baby.

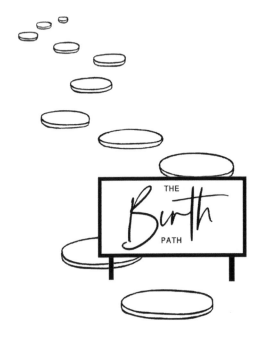

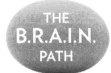

Preparing to bring new life into the world is like a path made up of stepping stones. Each step you take towards educating yourself in advance leads you closer to knowing what to expect, and knowing how to handle anything that crosses your path on the day. All paths contain the stepping stones to achieving a successful hypnobirth, no matter which path you choose or which path chooses you.

The important thing to be fully aware of at this moment is that you have now started an incredible journey here today. You are definitely on the right track by exploring the wonders of hypnobirthing. By taking each and every day to calm your mind and relax your body whenever you need, you will become an expert in emotional control, and in turn you will remain calm and relaxed when it is time for you to meet your precious baby.

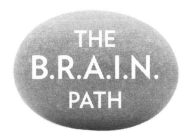

Where have your **BELIEFS** surrounding childbirth come from? When you **REFLECT** on your thoughts, memories and beliefs it affects the way you feel. What you put your **ATTENTION** and focus on is what you are more likely to attract into your life. The **INDIVIDUALS** you choose to be around can affect the way you feel and think. The **NEWS** and media can also affect the way you feel and think, especially when you are pregnant because you are naturally paying close attention to anything that might affect you or your baby.

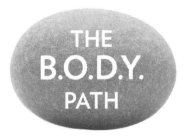

The B.O.D.Y. Path is about physically and emotionally **BONDING** with your baby. When you are breathing in fresh, nourishing oxygen your baby is too. **OXYGEN** is vital for your body to function effectively and efficiently. Have you ever wondered how incredibly well **DESIGNED** your body actually is? **YOU** and any fears you have can get in the way. This is something you will want to address.

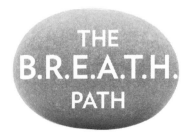

Knowing how to **BREATHE** the hypnobirthing way will get you through one of the most important days of your life. The hypnobirthing **RELAXATION** techniques will keep you calm, relaxed and in control, and creating a nurturing **ENVIRONMENT** will help you feel safe and secure. Knowing when and how to **APPLY** your hypnobirthing techniques is vital, alongside making time to **TRAIN** and to practise. **HORMONES** play a major part in the birth process so you will need to understand how they work too.

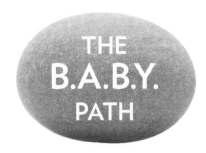

BIRTH PLANNING the hypnobirthing way is the first part of the B.A.B.Y. Path. It is important to know what the **ALTERNATIVES** are when making decisions about your baby's birth. Knowing what to pack in your **BIRTHING BAG** can make all the difference to how you feel when you give birth. I have included other considerations towards the end of the B.A.B.Y. Path because it is important that you know **Y – WHY.** You will need to consider these suggestions too.

'There are no guarantees that your birth will be pain-free. I do know it's possible though because mine was, and since becoming a hypnotherapist, teacher, trainer and doula I have had the privilege of witnessing many pain-free births.. It might feel like there is a lot for you to learn as you prepare for your baby's birth. In this book I will guide you through the basics in a way that's easy to understand so that you and your birth partner can start to feel more positive and look forward to your very special day.'

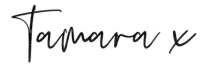

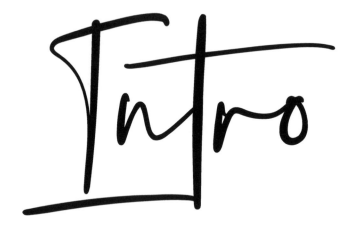

An Introduction to Hypnobirthing

Chapter 1:

Every Birth Is Unique

Hypnobirthing is a modern name for something that has always existed.

Some women instinctively birth by closing their eyes, going within, getting in the zone, blocking out the rest of the world and focusing, feeling and connecting purely on their baby moving down the birth path. They believe in themselves, their bodies and the birthing process, and seemingly just do it with a real sense of ease.

For others, a lack of knowledge, negative conditioning, birth trauma and fear can get in the way, negatively impacting the birthing process. This is a big problem, and where there is a problem there must be a solution. If you are feeling scared, anxious or even petrified about birthing your baby then hypnobirthing is an ideal solution for you.

The Birth Path will guide you every step of the way and provide you with a great foundation of information to support any hypnobirthing course. What if your baby needs to take an alternative route on the day? Hypnobirthing gives you the tools you need to cope with every type of birth.

There may be times when unexpected twists and turns play a part in the birth process causing a change of direction: knowing you have the necessary tools to cope in any situation will help you make calm and confident decisions along the way. Paths can change suddenly, so the more knowledge and tools you have in your 'hypnobirthing bag' the easier you and your partner will handle whatever happens on the day.

Hypnobirthing is a great birth choice

I've been chilling out in the hypnobirthing world since 2007 when my passion for wanting to make education better for all was ignited. What drives this passion of mine the most is knowing that the classes you choose to attend during your pregnancy will directly affect the outcome of your birth experience.

I know that learning hypnobirthing techniques will prevent you from having to go through what I had to endure during the traumatic birth of my first child. I will, of course, spare you the gory details; sharing will add no real value to your experience. You are unique, and that was my birth story, not yours.

What I do know is that this trauma could have been avoided if I had received better education at the time, but I also know I wouldn't be here now sharing this invaluable knowledge with you if I hadn't gone through what I did on that day. It was the scariest day of my life, although not just for me. It all started the very same day the Twin Towers went down in New York.

It took me many years and many tears to make peace with Frankie's birth, and it was definitely the fear that surrounded me on that very day that affected the way I was feeling. I remember being surrounded by shocking conversations and news reports as the atrocities of that day unfolded before my eyes.

'Am I really bringing a baby into a safe world? I can't do this. I'm not strong enough. It hurts too much, you've hurt my baby… where are you taking my baby?'

That day ended with me staring up into the eyes of many masked strangers. It was truly horrible. My mind and body together had decided that it wasn't a safe place for a baby to come out. I remember feeling completely out of control with a cascade of interventions that could have been avoided if I had prepared and educated myself better beforehand. I didn't know how to stand up for myself and neither did my husband. I don't blame him. Like many first-timers we had put our trust in the free NHS classes to educate us in the right way.

It took me a long time to recover from Frankie's birth and forgive myself for not having the foresight to know what now seems so obvious in hindsight. That experience made me who I am, and I am so pleased to be able to share that wisdom with you now as you embark on your unique pregnancy journey.

I am, however, happy to share in detail my positive hypnobirthing story of my second child, which you will find towards the back of this book. All stories featured within this book are from parents with whom I have been fortunate to cross paths on my journey as a hypnobirthing teacher and trainer.

Come with me now to the first day of spring 2007…

After achieving the most incredible hypnobirth with my daughter Alana on the first day of spring in 2007, I instantly (and I mean even before my milk came in) transformed into a woman possessed. I was inexorable! That means stubborn by the way – don't worry, I had to look it up too (let's reframe that… driven)! I was determined and focused on a mission to change the way pregnant couples prepared for this amazing moment!

I didn't even question the complexity or vastness of the task ahead because it just felt right. Could I do it single-handed? Not a chance. Was I going to give it my best shot? Yes, just you try and hold me back! Nothing could hold me back.

This feeling is common amongst hypnobirthing parents who become teachers. It is not a profession you go into for the money, even though many teachers are very successful. It's the knowledge that when a pregnant couple prepares well and equips themselves with the tools to cope with labour, their birth outcome will be calmer and much more satisfying for all involved.

Have you ever been so determined to make something happen that nothing and nobody could stand in your way?

I remember feeling the burning desire to shout from the rooftops that birth could be amazing after I did it. It was consuming my whole being and I couldn't make it stop. I was evangelistic in a sense like I had never been about anything else in my life before.

Every conversation I seemed to have somehow turned to birth, and I'm talking every conversation: with my mechanic, dentist, hairdresser, florist, accountant etc. I'm sure many thought I was crazy but I didn't care. I was a woman on a mission to reach out to as many people as I could about this life-changing knowledge that I had stumbled across purely by chance. I had discovered something truly amazing that the world needed to hear.

I often talk about the power of a surge (you may know that as a contraction) and how it can feel like an unstoppable force of nature, like your body has gone into automatic pilot, and so did the urge to dedicate my time to spreading the hypnobirthing message far and wide. Has dedicating such a big part of my life to teaching and training others to teach paid off? Right here, right now, it has because you are reading this book. One birth at a time, slowly but surely, myself and my hypnobirthing colleagues – who also share my passion for promoting top-quality education – are spreading the word out there because we know that it can make all the difference to the way you birth, particularly how you feel about your baby's birth afterwards.

Even though I had a newborn to look after I took immediate action to change the face of antenatal education. By the time Alana was six months old I had completed my training and was ready to teach. I am so pleased to say that this book is the result of my dedication and experience, having trained hundreds of hypnobirthing teachers and shared my wisdom with thousands of hypnobirthing families along the way.

I am so very proud of what I have achieved to date, and this book represents my life as a hypnobirthing mum, preacher, teacher, trainer, doula and the knowledge and wisdom that I have collected up to this point. This book represents where I believe hypnobirthing is right now. May it continue to grow and evolve to become even more popular and accessible for pregnant couples all over the world.

You will hear parts of my personal story throughout this book because in order to communicate anything, I have to reference it from a previous experience. It is how my brain works. I will be sharing my personal views and experiences with you throughout, but I am always mindful and aware that I am writing this book for you as well as providing a great resource to accompany any hypnobirthing course.

I am far from a closed book and I like to think that hypnobirthing has in fact brought me out of my shell somewhat with my total no holds barred openness to share the joys of birthing with anyone who crosses my path. No apologies – I can't help it. It is pure passion for what I do.

I have never done anything that felt so right before. I do have a medical background having trained and worked as a nurse, but this feeling was different. I had experienced what many people describe as their calling. I have found my true purpose, what I have been put here to do, and I know I am not alone in feeling this way.

Most, if not all, hypnobirthing teachers share this passion and that is why we do what we do. How can educating new parents so that they can bring their baby into the world in the best possible way not be one of the best jobs in the world? To me it is the best, and the most important job on the planet!

My hypnobirthing background

I taught the Mongan Method of HypnoBirthing for almost seven years as this was the programme I used for the birth of my daughter, Alana. Marie Mongan, my mentor, saw how dedicated to HypnoBirthing I was, so invited me to become Chair of UK HypnoBirthing. What a privilege it was to be asked and of course I obliged.

In this role I organised events for teachers so that we could all come together and celebrate the wonderful work we all did. Marie was affectionately known to many of us teachers as Mickey. Sadly she died in June 2019, and what a legacy she has entrusted us with. She will always be the inspirational woman who coined the phrase HypnoBirthing.

'When you change the way you view birth, the way you birth will change.' – Marie Mongan

Birth is a unique experience for every woman

Being a hypnobirthing teacher and doula is a rewarding journey: one of mysteries, excitement and of course many elements of surprise. I will never know everything and neither will any other hypnobirthing teacher or birth worker because each birth is unique, like a snowflake, and just when you think you've seen it all you are very quickly reminded that you never will.

Even though I taught Mickey's method for many years, I felt there was always another hidden depth that needed to be revealed and built on. It was an American programme and it wasn't specific enough to the way women were birthing in the UK. Many of her techniques were focused primarily on birth and not so much on becoming tools for life afterwards. This was important to me. Being in the position to which Mickey had appointed me meant that the majority of the hypnobirthing community knew who I was: outspoken, passionate and one to represent hypnobirthing at every opportunity.

I found myself getting to know many UK teachers and before long I had found myself in a position of influence. Hypnobirthing needed to change and I was going to be the one to do it. I saw my role as the person who was going to increase awareness of hypnobirthing, and in doing so I knew I needed to give this education and our teaching materials the facelift that teachers here in the UK were eagerly awaiting.

I shared with other teachers how I taught hypnobirthing, how I would never set women up for failure or disappointment, how I never promised a pain-free birth and how I made classes fun and interactive. I knew that it was vital to really promote how this education can be used no matter what turn your birthing takes on the day, which is the true value and essence of hypnobirthing. I regularly welcomed other hypnobirthing teachers and midwives into my classes so they could learn from me, and I was always happy to support them in any way I could.

I made hypnobirthing modern and fresh again, but this time not only did it get a new look it got a new name. It was time to shake up the hypnobirthing world and make a bold statement.

It was time to make hypnobirthing stand out and be recognised as an incredibly life-changing way to birth. In 2013, I launched a new hypnobirthing programme and called it The Wise Hippo Birthing Programme®. Everything evolves and that's a healthy thing; it was my job to make sure that hypnobirthing continued to grow in the right direction.

Congratulations on finding hypnobirthing too

At this point, I would like to congratulate you on your pregnancy and for finding *The Birth Path*. It's going to be a journey of discovery and thank you for not burying your head in the sand like some pregnant couples do. Your baby will be coming out soon so you need to know what to expect and I'm sure you don't want to witness your birth partner being caught like a rabbit in the headlights either.

One of the most important aspects of hypnobirthing is learning how the mind works. This is fundamental when it comes to acknowledging the importance of mental health and the wellbeing of the mother as this can impact all future relationships. Think about that for a moment. Today we live in an era where mental health is being taken more seriously than ever, with the Royal Family raising awareness, and the media giving it centre stage.

Hypnobirthing teachers love what they do

Hypnobirthing teachers who have birthed using the techniques for themselves, or have witnessed first-hand others using these techniques, know that birth can be a truly empowering experience. This is why it is important for you to also watch some hypnobirths either online or in class. Your hypnobirthing teacher will enjoy sharing inspiring birth footage from her collection in class of other mums using these techniques. There is nothing more powerful to help shift your mindset than witnessing for yourself women using hypnobirthing techniques and how their birth partners support them with that; after all, seeing is believing!

I will be referring to your teacher as 'her' throughout this book as I have only ever trained one male hypnobirthing teacher before; a father of three and a fireman who teaches classes together with his wife in Australia.

I trust that you will find a supportive teacher who is just right for you, either now or after you have devoured this book inside and out. I know this because the teachers who thrive in this industry do so because they are completely dedicated to providing you with an enormous amount of value. It is impossible to put a price on a positive birth experience but if I had to give you a figure it would be in the millions.

Is it possible to hypnobirth without learning from a teacher?

There is more than one hypnobirthing programme on the market, some are online and some are face to face. If you live in an area that doesn't have a hypnobirthing teacher then you can do an online course as this book will support any online hypnobirthing course. I'm personally not a fan of online learning; I am not disciplined enough and I'm easily distracted. If that sounds familiar then a face-to-face course is definitely for you. Lives are busy and hypnobirthing needs commitment in order to get the best results. Scheduling time specifically for birth preparation is a great way to ensure that you and your partner are both working together, opening up conversations about what is important to you both and maintaining that you are both on the same page. This will be much more achievable with the support of a hypnobirthing teacher to guide you and your birth partner along the way.

'I've done it both ways; online and face to face. I didn't really have the money to spend on a face-to-face class with my first and it now has to be one of my biggest regrets. I know this because when I booked a hypnobirthing class with my second baby it was the relationship and support I received from my teacher and her reassurance that helped me achieve an amazing birth. Doing it alone takes the fun out of it. My partner would get fidgety and fall asleep so not really sure how much he got out of the online course. There were some parts online that I really couldn't understand so I was often left confused.' Lauren, Hertfordshire, UK

Hypnobirthing is spreading slowly but surely…

Even though some proactive NHS trusts have now implemented hypnobirthing into their antenatal offerings making it more mainstream, it is still early days as the most common reason I receive for them not teaching it is primarily down to government funding issues. What a shame!

My dream is that after reading this book and attending a hypnobirthing course you will transform into a confident and empowered parent who achieves the right birth on the day for you and your baby. One of the best parts about being a hypnobirthing teacher is that heart-warming moment when you receive the exciting birth news from someone you have taught. The hypnobirthing community relies highly on parents sharing their inspiring stories as this helps spread the word, and we cannot thank them enough for this; how can we share positive birth stories if they're all kept a secret! As previously mentioned, I know you will thoroughly enjoy hearing and watching their birth footage in class.

Sometimes the smallest step in the right direction ends up being the biggest step of your life

I tried so hard to change the 'hypnobirthing' name but in the end it prevailed. As the Founder of The Wise Hippo Birthing Programme®, the techniques that I personally choose to teach in my classes are the Wise Hippo techniques because of how effective and easy they are to implement into your everyday life. That is not to say that other hypnobirthing programmes are any less effective. As far as I am concerned, it all comes down to the teacher, their dedication and how they show up for you. As a hypnobirthing teacher trainer, I am fully committed to making sure that my teachers receive the best training, products and support.

When I launched this programme in 2013, hypnobirthing was not as popular as it is today, so changing the name felt like a wise idea at the time. The Wise Hippo community has played a huge part in raising the profile of hypnobirthing in the antenatal education market, and for that I am so grateful for the wonderful teachers who work tirelessly to make birth education better for all.

The word hypnobirthing rolls off people's tongues. It is now a recognised birth choice, it's what the media call it, it's what celebrities endorse, and it's how most people describe what hypnosis for childbirth is. Even England football captain and Wise Hippo dad Harry Kane tweeted that his daughter was a hypnobirthed baby. If hypnosis features in a birthing programme it is likely that it will be described as hypnobirthing, and it is for this reason that this unusual sounding word is here to stay.

The hypnobirthing reputation

I believe that reputation is one of the most important assets for a product as it signals to customers whether or not it can be trusted with their time, energy, and money. Customer experience is all about attention to detail as this is what will encourage you to recommend this type of education after your hypnobirth.

Good customer experience is a great way to encourage positive word of mouth which is what hypnobirthing teachers thrive and rely on. Giving your teacher feedback on their classes is important as it ensures that your teacher will be offering you the very best experience they can. By doing this you will be playing an important role yourself; ensuring that hypnobirthing continues to receive the great reputation that it undoubtedly deserves.

Feedback also helps strengthen the product by keeping it relevant and modern. A happy hypnobirthing experience is what will encourage more and more couples to spread the word far and wide. Hypnobirthing teachers do not take this for granted and are constantly searching for ways to keep their classes current and enjoyable.

There is, of course, plenty of healthy competition out there today with NCT and NHS classes and it's great that there is this choice available. I know some wonderful midwives who teach NHS classes and some equally wonderful NCT teachers; but not all teachers are good at what they do so please be mindful of this and ensure that you thoroughly check out their credentials first.

The hypnobirthing community comes together annually to celebrate

In celebration of all the wonderful work that hypnobirthing teachers do, I launched the very first World Hypnobirthing Day on 21st March 2019 (my daughter Alana's birthday) and it was incredible. Hypnobirthing teachers and parents from all over the world came together to celebrate by hosting coffee mornings and other events. I collaborated with leaders from other hypnobirthing programmes on this special day and together we recorded a beautiful meditation for all. I am looking forward to doing it all again in years to come and I invite you to join in the celebrations too.

Finally we are starting to understand what hypnobirthing really is

Hypnobirthing has come a long way since I birthed my daughter and it's great to see that so many more pregnant couples are looking into it as a serious option. This book will clarify what hypnobirthing is and what it can and cannot do for you. I am sure you and your hypnobirthing teacher will enjoy the information I have put together for you within *The Birth Path*.

It has taken many years to persuade our NHS midwives that hypnobirthing can reduce their intervention rates, birth trauma and improve the mental health of birthing women. I am so happy to say that the hard work has paid off because over the last few years I have witnessed an increase in midwives who are training to become hypnobirthing teachers, many of whom I have trained myself, really showing how much they are recognising the benefits of this wonderful option.

The evidence of how much it helps a woman in labour is right before their eyes and it is too powerful to ignore. It is a fact that hypnobirthing helps parents to achieve the right birth on the day; a phrase we use often in The Wise Hippo Birthing Programme. Today the majority of midwives have heard of hypnobirthing even if they don't quite understand what it is… yet.

The word hypnobirthing intrigues people and I am often asked to speak at events to share more about what it entails, and more importantly, the benefits of birthing this way. I have heard people suggest it sounds hippy, airy fairy, esoteric and alternative, just to mention a few, but this is happening less and less. If you value great antenatal education then hypnobirthing is for you.

You must remain sceptical of your scepticism

I have often thought that the name 'hypnobirthing' can make it sound like something that it isn't, and if we simply reframe the word and replace it with relaxation instead it can feel more palatable for those who feel a little uncomfortable with not knowing what it is.

I was pretty sceptical when I first heard of hypnobirthing, and my husband Serg was even more so, particularly when we were told to consider renaming the word 'CONTRACTION' with his name 'SURGE'… that just felt really weird! Of course, up to this point we only knew what we knew and that was what happened during our son Frankie's birth, so hearing that it was possible for birth to be completely opposite to this experience was challenging. It is pretty normal to be faced with a sceptical mum or birth partner as a teacher; I secretly love watching the transformation unfold class by class. The penny usually drops at the end of the first class when couples realise that hypnobirthing is based on science and medical fact. Explaining the science behind it all is the real mindset converter. Sadly there are still many examples in the media that misrepresent hypnobirthing or portray it in a certain way, leaving behind a disappointed new mum who may feel like her much anticipated hypnobirth had failed. We teach the skills and tools to manage birth no matter what happens on the day. Unfortunately we can't control the media (only provide couples with the tools to discern and protect themselves from any negativity).

'I remember watching a hypnobirthing mum in labour on the TV programme "One Born Every Minute", and of course it ended with her screaming for pain relief thus making a mockery of her birth preferences and hypnobirthing. The media, of course, set hypnobirthing up as promising her a pain-free, natural birth.'

Tamara x

Let me tell you here and now, no reputable hypnobirthing teacher would ever promise you or anyone else a pain-free birth.

It is definitely not all doom and gloom with the media, because there are many of those in the limelight who continue to credit hypnobirthing for helping them achieve a positive birth experience and the list is growing. Here are some well-known names that I'm sure you'll recognise: Kate Middleton, Duchess of Cambridge, Meghan Markle, Duchess of Sussex, Jessica Alba, Pamela Anderson, Kate Kane (wife of footballer Harry Kane), Russell Brand, Fearne Cotton, *The Only Way is Essex* mums including Ferne McCann, Sam Faiers and Danielle Armstrong, Tom and Giovanna Fletcher (I remember Tom likening hypnobirthing to 'Jedi birthing' when interviewed. Love that!), *Britain's Got Talent* judge Alesha Dixon, TV personality and 'Loose Woman'

Nadia Sawalha, and Angelina Jolie with her planned Caesarean birth. Yes, you can still use hypnobirthing if you require a Caesarean birth as the skills are transferable to any type of birth. More on that later on.

It is obvious from Harry Kane's Instagram post that they achieved the right birth on the day. If Harry can make the time in his sporting schedule to attend a Wise Hippo course to prepare, then I am sure your partner can too.

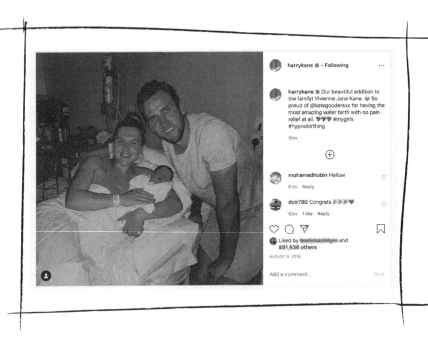

Chapter 2:

Learning Tools For Life

I have taught hypnobirthing to many midwives, including many NHS trusts, which has definitely contributed to the acceptance of the hypnobirthing name. The dedication and hard work of these passionate midwives has supported hypnobirthing to become even more widely accepted by mainstream society.

They have waded their way through all the red tape, the powers that be, and the tight purse strings to make it happen. I applaud them. Seeing midwives teach and support hypnobirthing within an NHS trust is my dream come true.

The NHS trusts that have brought in hypnobirthing as an option for their pregnant couples have done so because they hold it in such high regard. It initiates a powerful education and supports mental health and wellbeing.

How can pregnancy affect mental health?

I have included the following information from The Royal College of Psychiatrists[1] because becoming more aware of the importance of your mental health and wellbeing – particularly whilst pregnant – and preparing to become a mother, will enable you to create the best possible environment within which to nurture your unborn baby, so that they, too, can benefit from this knowledge and become a relaxed and loved little individual.

Pregnancy is often a very happy and exciting time. But not every woman feels this way. You may have mixed, or even negative, feelings about being pregnant. You may find it more difficult than others to cope with the changes and uncertainties that pregnancy brings. Many things can affect how you feel in pregnancy. These include physical symptoms (e.g. morning sickness), the support you have (or don't have), and any events you find stressful.

You might be worrying about how you will cope with pregnancy or having a baby. It's normal to feel stressed or anxious at times. It is natural to worry about:

- The changes in your role (becoming a mother, pausing your career).

- The changes in your relationships.

- Whether you will be a good parent.

- Fear that there will be problems with your pregnancy or your baby.

- Physical health problems and pregnancy complications.

- Fear of childbirth.

- Lack of support and feeling alone.

1 https://www.rcpsych.ac.uk/mental-health/treatments-and-wellbeing/mental-health-in-pregnancy#faq-accoridon-collap, November 2018

As many as one in five women experiences mental health issues in pregnancy or after birth. It can happen to anyone. Depression and anxiety are the most common issues in pregnancy. These affect about 10 to 15 out of every 100 pregnant women.

How your mental health is affected during pregnancy depends on many things. These may include:

- Any existing mental health issues.

- Stopping medication for a mental health problem.

- Recent stressful events in your life.

- How you feel about your pregnancy – you may or may not be happy about being pregnant.

- Upsetting memories about difficulties in your own childhood.

You may have anxious or negative thoughts about your pregnancy or your baby. You may find changes in your weight and body shape or size difficult (particularly if you have ever suffered from an eating disorder). Sometimes symptoms caused by your pregnancy can be confused with symptoms of poor mental health. For example, broken sleep and lack of energy are common in both pregnancy and depression.

To find out more about mental health in pregnancy please visit www.rcpsych.ac.uk

Ever heard the phrase, 'It takes a village to raise a child'?

Let's explore how this can affect you. It's imperative that as a new mum you feel seen, heard, and supported on your birth and parenting journey.

Start to create your village now. It's important. Grab a pen and paper and write down a few suggestions as to where you might find the type of people you value. This could mean moving closer to your parents, finding a good parenting network, connecting with positive online support networks, and not feeling pressured to go back to work before you're ready. It is for this very reason that so many hypnobirthing mums become hypnobirthing teachers themselves afterwards. Sharing the parenting and work arrangements as a couple may also be an option for some, but, of course, there may be financial implications involved here.

There is a large disconnect in the messages we are given by society about becoming a parent. We are bombarded by idyllic parenting images on social media: mothers who seamlessly seem to juggle work, marriage, children, exercise and a perfect home and endless childhood accomplishments. In our own minds we have this idea that there is a perfect way to parent. There isn't.

'I remember the words used by my husband when I was once in a complete state of overwhelm with a three-month-old baby. In a calm voice he simply said, 'There is no trophy, Tamara'. So why was I behaving like there was? He was so right! A simple sentence, so profound and so true. Conditioning is a strong force to be reckoned with. Your hypnobirthing teacher will help you break your negative patterns of behaviour.'

Tamara x

Trying to juggle too much could negatively impact your relationship with your partner and your child. Ask for help or reprioritise.

It's common for a couple to meet online and live far away from their home roots. Occasionally visits from lifelong friends or family don't go far enough. The stress of having to raise children without the support of a village, in conjunction with the stress of trying to balance so many other things, can leave parents feeling like they are not coping. The hypnobirthing techniques you learn in class will become your tools for life; they will support you well whenever you feel you are not coping. Use them often.

If living near family is not a feasible option, consider which trusted friends can become your village. Create authentic relationships based on trust and be honest about what your struggles are. Being there for one another is how we reclaim our village. You may even find that the other pregnant couples you meet in your hypnobirthing course will become lifelong friends..

Parents who master the art of decreasing stress are better able to utilise parenting skills. Consider your life and think about ways that you can simplify it. This could mean cutting back on certain activities, making sure family dinners happen regularly and prioritising sleep for the entire family.

It may be a case of reaching out to a parenting specialist or a therapist. This may be the perfect catalyst for helping you to reclaim your priorities. Many hypnobirthing teachers also have these skills, and if they don't they will know someone who will. Parenting is challenging and there is no such thing as a perfect parent.

Asking for help from someone you can trust is a sign of wisdom not weakness!

'Pregnancy is a time of profound physical and psychological change. The transition to motherhood can be complex and difficult, and in all the discourse about pregnancy and birth, the huge personal changes that women undergo can be overlooked. In the 21st century it can seem that mothers are blamed and blame themselves for everything, as they struggle to manage their multiple identities as mothers, lovers, sisters and daughters. The book "Why Mothering Matters" is a nuanced and revealing discussion of how it can feel to become a mother in modern society. It calls for better recognition of the work of motherhood, and better support for women and families as they learn what parenting looks like for them'. Maddie McMahon[2] *(Maddie was my doula teacher in 2008)*

Hypnobirthing will NOT promise that your birth will be pain-free or that it will ever happen in a certain way

If you come across a teacher who guarantees that hypnobirthing will give you a pain-free birth, walk away. She is not the right teacher for you. If she is

2 McMahon, Maddie; *Why Mothering Matters*; Pinter & Martin Ltd; 25 October 2018 (1st edition)

adamant that your birth will go a certain way, run away. She is definitely not the teacher for you unless of course she has an authentic crystal ball. If you know where I can find one of those let me know!

As a passionate hypnobirthing teacher, my face-to-face classes have always focused on the right birth on the day, not a pain-free birth without drugs or intervention because let's be real, birth is unpredictable, but you can take the reins and choose how to respond and hypnobirthing will show you how. As a teacher and birth doula, I have witnessed the best laid plans go out the window, and been honoured to support the couple in that moment to embrace a new direction.

 It is possible to have a pain-free birth. I had one with my daughter, and I have many birth stories from my mums and teachers who have enjoyed pain-free and even ecstatic births. I have even had the privilege of filming these births too which I would love to share with you. There is a lot of power in knowing that birth can be comfortable and enjoyed even if I cannot promise it. You can expect a better birth when you become an expert in relaxation, and that's what hypnobirthing aims to achieve.

I have dedicated a whole section of this book to talking about pain because it is important that you understand it. No hypnobirthing teacher should ever shy away from talking about pain in their classes, particularly when it is one of the main reasons why so many women turn to hypnobirthing in the first place.

We can thank the media for spreading the rumour that hypnobirthing results in a pain-free birth. I for one have never heard any teacher promise this and I trust I never will. Saying that hypnobirthing results in a pain-free birth attracts attention and that is the likely reason why the media have connected the two like this. I suppose what it could do is encourage couples to look into it further, but it could also set women up for failure and disappointment when their birth doesn't go this way. A positive birth experience is more likely to occur, however, once you become an expert in relaxation after attending a hypnobirthing course, that's for sure.

Remember, good education can change anyone. A good teacher can change everything.

Why this hypnobirthing book is different

This book can be utilised alongside any hypnobirthing course (not exclusively The Wise Hippo). It is designed to be a great resource for teachers and expectant couples. This book is a modern approach to hypnobirthing with up-to-date information based on the way hypnobirthing is currently viewed, and how it has progressed and evolved up to this point in time.

The Birth Path is based on facts and evidence as well as the many years of experience and research I have conducted working with parents-to-be and other hypnobirthing teachers. I have lived and breathed hypnobirthing since I discovered it. I hope you find this book to be one of the most valuable pieces of literature you will read during your pregnancy.

There are plenty of birthing books on the shelf. I am sure you will agree that there is much information out there, some of which is conflicting.In this book you will find references to what I believe to be the best material to support your hypnobirth.

I have met some truly incredible teachers over the years, many of whom have never even taught my programme and I would not think twice about recommending their services. It is the quality of the teacher, her passion, her credibility and her ethos that is fundamentally the most important thing when looking for your hypnobirthing teacher. What is her reputation like in your area? Have you researched the services she can offer?

'My children have always done so much better at school when they respect and like their teachers. They have always received higher results in subjects with teachers who enjoy their job and are passionate about teaching. For this reason it is important to find a teacher who is just right for you so that you can connect with her in the same way too.'

Tamara x

Your hypnobirthing teacher will pave the way for you

The great news is that there are many passionate influencers out there dedicating their lives to making birthing better. As far as I am concerned, it all starts with the education you choose, and there is no better way than attending a hypnobirthing course with a passionate hypnobirthing teacher to guide and support you and your birth partner.

Have I mentioned how important your birth partner is yet? There is a whole section dedicated to the role of your birth partner; no more twiddling thumbs or texting! Your hypnobirthing teacher will equip your birth partner, who has a very specific role to play on the day, with a tool bag (not the hammer and nail kind) which will help them gain the knowledge to support you with confidence and knowhow.

Attending a face-to-face hypnobirthing course with your partner is highly effective

Hypnobirthing teachers primarily receive bookings through word of mouth so ask around and see what teacher others are recommending in your area. It's important that what they share and promote resonates with you so check out their websites, social media feeds, reviews etc. Remember to trust yourself to make a good choice. What resonates with one person might not resonate with another. To find the best teacher for you, trust your instincts and your heart alongside any research.

Hypnobirthing teachers are special people with a wealth of knowledge that will open your mind to the possibilities that birth can be an enjoyable experience and one to be cherished forever. Teaching hypnobirthing is one of the most rewarding jobs on the planet, that's for sure, and I am sure the teacher that you find to support you will totally agree with that!

Your hypnobirthing teacher does not need to have a medical background, be a qualified midwife or doula or even a hypnotherapist (even though many of them are). The primary role of a hypnobirthing teacher is to teach you how to become an expert in relaxation and empower you and your birth partner with the tools and knowledge to help you make informed choices and decisions during your pregnancy and on your birthing day.

It is not their role to make any medical decisions for you but they will help you to understand how to make informed decisions that are right for you and your baby.

My main objective in compiling the information contained within this book is to make sure that no matter what hypnobirthing course or teacher you choose to teach you, this information will be a supportive resource for you that will provide you with a wonderful foundation, whatever hypnobirthing course you choose to attend.

Face-to-face communication allows for better rapport and trust-building than audio or written communications, which can make all the difference in achieving the best possible birth outcome for you.

Like anything, you could find most of the information you'd need on the internet for free. But it would take you hours (and you don't know exactly what you are looking for). You might miss out on:

• Human connection – hypnobirthing teachers are great at reading body language and can pick up on things that you may not even be aware of consciously.

• You can never underestimate the power of physical presence in terms of learning. Hypnobirthing teachers know how to teach all learning types (did you know there are many different ways to learn and your mind will have a preference for one or two of them).

• No question is a silly question! You will be able to ask any questions that are specific to your individual needs with an instant response.

- You will feel supported throughout your entire pregnancy knowing that you can contact your teacher at any time, providing you with reassurance and continuity of care throughout.

- A midwife colleague once said to me, 'I love hypnobirthing because it means that someone is genuinely invested in you as a real person, not just a number.'

- A hypnobirthing course will provide peer support as well as being a special place to build new friendships with others who are expecting at the same time as you. Often the couples you meet in a hypnobirthing course become friends for life.

- A hypnobirthing course, whether it be private or in a group setting, will be tailored to each class. Teachers are aware that whilst they follow a particular structure, no two classes are ever the same.

- Your important questions may go unanswered in an online course and this can be detrimental in terms of your progress. Your teacher needs to follow your progress and celebrate your transformational journey with you.

- Connection and continuity of support. Your hypnobirthing teacher will nurture you and if you like hugs there will be plenty coming your way.

- Not all pregnancies are straightforward so hypnobirthing classes can be tailored to your specific needs.

- Hypnobirthing teachers continually update their knowledge which is vital in this fast-paced, changing world. Hospital policies change and new research is always coming out. It is important that you are made aware of what is going on in your area right now.

- Your hypnobirthing teacher will check in with you often to see if you are practising enough. In order for this knowledge and particularly the techniques to become second nature to you, having a disciplined approach is crucial. Your teacher will give you a gentle nudge of encouragement in the right direction if need be. Having someone to be accountable to is often the most effective way to achieve the best results.

Reading about hypnobirthing won't make you any better at it, just like reading a book about singing doesn't turn you into a brilliant vocalist. What you need in order to be confident and competent in hypnobirthing is practice and regular time with a teacher who observes your progress along the way.

'I got lucky, really lucky, because if I hadn't overheard the conversation between other mums talking about doulas when I was pregnant I would have never looked into it. I am sure you agree the word "doula" is a strange word but once I had Googled it for myself it all just seemed so obvious. I needed a doula but to meet one who introduced me to hypnobirthing, well it couldn't have been better than that. Thank you Suzanne Howlett – you crossed my path at the perfect time!'

Tamara x

Babies come down the 'birth path' not the 'birth canal'

Have you ever wondered why certain words can make you feel a particular way? I've been saying that babies come down the 'birth path' for well over 10 years now because it sounds so much nicer than the more commonly used phrase 'birth canal'.

When it's time for your baby to be born they will come down the birth path to meet you, unless of course they decide to take an alternate path. I'm not sure about you but the word 'canal' makes me think of something completely different. In fact when I asked my 12-year-old daughter Alana what the word 'canal' meant to her she replied 'a river type thingy' which is pretty much what I was thinking too. So there you have it! Your baby will be coming down the birth path to meet you rather than the birth canal and I'm sure you'll agree it's a softer, more positive use of language.

Now I know that sometimes babies have other ideas and can decide on a different route, which can involve twists, turns, humps and bumps along the way, so my question to you is, if your baby does unexpectedly take a different path, how are you going to deal with that? I am sure you will agree that just like everything in life where there is more than one way to do something, there is also more than one way to birth your baby. So, whether your baby is born vaginally or via a Caesarean birth, the knowledge gained within *The Birth Path*, alongside your hypnobirthing course, will guide you towards a calmer and more positive birth experience. Achieving the right birth on the day is the most important thing on your birthing journey.

Hypnobirthing is a method of birthing

Hypnobirthing prides itself in offering the highest standard of education for birth preparation. It is an antenatal education programme that supports you and your birthing partner to prepare for your baby's birth in a way that feels right for you. Your physical, physiological and psychological health matters; now more than ever.

Hypnobirthing will help you understand the connection between your mind and your body, and how you can ensure that they are working together in the best possible way, for both your labour and your life in general. You will learn how to relax emotionally and physically and how to plan for success no matter what path your birthing takes.

Along with practical birth planning, your birth partner's role, physical preparations for birth and so much more, you can be sure that you are receiving the best possible education on how to birth your baby feeling calm, relaxed and in control when you attend a hypnobirthing course.

Chapter 3:

Empowering You And Your Birth Partner

Every woman, every baby and every birth is different and your hypnobirthing teacher will help you to prepare for the birth that you'd like to have whilst ensuring that you have the skills to adapt calmly and confidently should you need to deviate from that.

Your hypnobirthing course should be simple to understand and the practice enjoyable, enabling you to easily integrate it into your everyday life. You are learning skills not only for birth, but also for life. Whilst hypnobirthing focuses on birth being a natural event, I do not believe that it is anyone's right to dictate to any woman what their birth should be like. Your hypnobirthing teacher will therefore provide you and your birth partner with a non-judgemental learning environment.

The main focus of this education is on teaching you how to relax, breathe and trust your body to know what to do instinctively. Belief and trust create confidence, which is what is required on the day you birth your baby. Achieving a positive birth experience will be based on making informed choices and receiving as much information as you can to make your decisions. I believe that focusing on the 'best birth' you can imagine has many more benefits for all involved in the birthing process.

It is fair to say that no-one knows what birth you will have, but by focusing on the birth that you want, it is more likely to happen. If it doesn't, what you have learnt will help you make informed choices about every aspect of your baby's birth ensuring that you and your baby have the right birth on the day. I hope that with this in mind it makes sense not to rehearse a negative outcome when you can enjoy focusing on a positive one. Your hypnobirthing teacher may ask you to focus on your best birth possible throughout your pregnancy to help you feel more positive.

'My experiences as a midwife have taught me that women's bodies still work. Here is your chance to be exposed to a new understanding of an ancient system of knowledge that you can add to your general understanding of what birth means. Wherever and however you intend to give birth, your experience will impact your emotions, your mind, your body, and your spirit for the rest of your life.' Ina May Gaskin[3]

Hypnobirthing gives you the ability to achieve the right birth for you and your baby no matter what happens on the day. Many hypnobirthing couples report low use of pain-relieving drugs and a low requirement for intervention; this is not, however, the goal. The most important thing is that all women feel that they had 'the right birth on the day' and of course I want that for you too. You will be in good hands with your chosen hypnobirthing teacher but please

3 Gaskin, Ina May; *Ina May's Guide to Childbirth*; Vermilion; 7 August 2008 (3rd edition)

ensure you have done your research first so that she is the perfect fit for you and your birth partner.

How does the hypnobirthing community view birth?

The ethos is focused primarily on choice. The hypnobirthing community believes that every woman has the right to be able to make an informed choice about how, when and where her baby is birthed. It is dedicated to empowering women and their birth partners so that they can achieve the best possible outcome for themselves and their babies.

You will be asked to focus on the best birth possible whilst appreciating that sometimes nature needs a helping hand. With this approach you will be able to look forward to your baby's birth without the concern that it needs to turn out a certain way to be deemed a successful birth.

A positive birth experience is a state of mind, it's not defined by what happens during labour and birth, but by how you feel about your baby's birth. Your hypnobirthing teacher will teach you skills and knowledge that will empower you to trust your instincts and ensure that you and your baby have the right birth on the day.

Is hypnobirthing suited to everyone?

Hypnobirthing is for everyone. All women are unique and hypnobirthing classes are designed to cater for individual needs. You will have your own concerns and aspirations for your baby's birth and will be looking for a birth preparation programme to suit you. Hypnobirthing will support whatever choices you make along the way and if your plans need to change your teacher will cover that too.

Hypnobirthing teachers will provide you with the knowledge to build your confidence so that you can instinctively know what is right for you and your baby, and will therefore not offer their own opinions on what they believe you should or should not do. Your hypnobirthing teacher will be non-judgemental in her approach to teaching you.

Your hypnobirthing teacher will activate and open your mind to new possibilities, curiosity, wisdom and knowledge, so brace yourself as it's time to start your transformational journey, and your teacher will be by your side guiding you every step of the way. The destination being, you guessed it, the right birth on the day!

There is not one right way to birth and I appreciate that there isn't one right way to prepare for birth either, only the right way for each individual woman and her partner. The main focus is, of course, to provide you with the support and tools to achieve the best birth possible no matter what type of birth you want to have.

Hypnobirthing isn't just about natural birth

There is an assumption that women only attend a hypnobirthing course because they want a natural birth without drugs. However, from my experience many women also attend classes because of their intense fear about how they are going to cope with labour.

What I have always found wonderful is that even women with the most extreme fear, who perhaps attend a course without any intention of saying no to the pain-relieving drugs, go down the route of not having any simply because they didn't need them, not because they had a strong desire to avoid them. If they do need drugs or intervention they know that is okay; it's about what's right for them. You will learn how to make the right decisions for yourself and your baby based on what happens and how you are feeling on the day. The hypnobirthing method is designed to relieve anxiety and build confidence in a way that will enable you to focus on your baby's birth in a manner that is right for you.

Feeling proud of your baby's birth no matter what happens on the day is what hypnobirthing will help you achieve.

Having a baby using hypnobirthing

Giving birth will probably be one of the most profound events in your life. During pregnancy, along with growing a healthy baby, your body is obviously preparing itself for birth. But this shouldn't be the only preparation. It is important for you to prepare emotionally and practically for the arrival of your baby too.

Considering what your birth may be like helps you and your birth partner to make your own plans and preparations, ensuring that you are not only clear about what kind of birth you want, but also how to cope with any changes that may take place. This includes knowing about your choices regarding where you will birth, who will be supporting you and what may happen if nature needs a helping hand.

What hypnobirthing offers parents

- The opportunity to feel prepared for your baby's birth, both emotionally and practically.

- Understanding of the physical and psychological processes that occur in the mother during labour and birth.

- Preparation for the role of birth partner. Partners have a very specific role to play.

- A sense of being ready to meet your baby and what to expect immediately after the birth.

- Alleviation of your fears, building confidence and belief in your ability to trust your instincts.

- The tools learnt will enable you to remain calm, relaxed and in control during your baby's birth no matter what path your birthing takes.

- Bonding together as a family.

Getting the most out of your hypnobirthing course

Much of what you know is learnt through repetition. You will find that I have deliberately covered the most important points more than once in this book and it has been written this way to ensure that I not only plant the seed but that it is able to grow. After all, repetition is the mother of all skills.

Repetition is a great way to learn, and when you are looking to make a change, this is achieved in the same way. By attending a course over a number of sessions you will not only have the opportunity to learn gradually in stages but your hypnobirthing teacher will also continually motivate you to practise. Attending several classes also allows the time to explore your feelings, relax with your partner and resolve and release any anxieties that may arise.

I recommend that your hypnobirthing teacher works with you personally and follows your progress, so that you can ensure that you are fully prepared, relaxed and confident as you approach the birth of your baby. For those who are late in pregnancy (37 weeks plus) and therefore attending over a shorter period of time, please be assured that you are still able to use the techniques successfully. I know this because I stumbled across hypnobirthing purely by chance at 36 weeks pregnant. It was knowing that I only had a month or so left that made me approach my preparation with 100% dedication right to the very end.

'Enjoying a coffee break and some fresh air whilst attending a hospital birth, I crossed paths with a young woman in labour pacing around the waiting room downstairs. She was looking rather distressed and not coping very well at all. I couldn't resist stepping in and providing her with some immediate reassurance and support.

I asked her to close her eyes and focus only on my voice. In between her surges that were roughly seven minutes apart I taught her all about her amazing body and how to breathe through her surges. I wasn't able to stay very long as my client needed me by her side but I knew that if she continued to do what I had taught her, she would start to get some control back.

It wasn't until the next day when I went to visit my client on the ward that I noticed her bed was right next to the lady I had met in the corridor. She couldn't thank me enough for teaching her how to breathe and focus, enabling her to get through each surge so much so that she said she didn't need any pain relief. She birthed her baby eight hours later on her hands and knees after our brief encounter. Don't you just love it when you happen to be in the right place at just the right time?

She shared that she kept her eyes closed pretty much the entire time and focused on her baby moving down just like I had taught her. Now that is the true power of hypnobirthing and a great example of how being taught even the smallest amount of the right education really can make all the difference.'

Tamara x

Is it ever too late to start hypnobirthing?

The motivation that comes from your birth being imminent cannot be underestimated, both in terms of your conscious desire to practice and your subconscious ability to absorb the new information. If other circumstances mean it is more beneficial for you to attend a compressed course, you may find that you need to practise with more discipline, since you will have a shorter period of face-to-face time with your hypnobirthing teacher. Hypnobirthing can be taught privately or in a group setting with other pregnant couples depending on your preference.

All pregnant women are different and so is the education out there!

All pregnancies are different and all women should be treated as individuals. Your needs are specific to your pregnancy and your needs will be specific to your labour. It seems that the majority of information given to pregnant couples often focuses on what can go wrong during labour and birth. You will read about the dreadful classes I attended as part of my own personal story at the back of this book. It is frustrating to see that not a lot has changed.

'I moved house in 2019 and throughout that process I met a few estate agents. One particular estate agent named Jack thoroughly enjoyed our chat about childbirth, having just become a father himself a month prior. I thought I would take the

opportunity to quiz him on the antenatal classes he attended and what they covered. He had attended the very same classes I did 18 years ago in the very same room.

I wasn't surprised to hear that not a lot had changed and that they were still passing around instruments in class, re-enacting Caesarean births and learning all about things that could go wrong. There was no talk of breathing or relaxation, let alone how the female body is designed to birth. He said that he and his partner felt even more unprepared and scared having attended these classes....I can still remember that feeling. At that moment I felt deflated; I had been teaching hypnobirthing for over 10 years but it seems these free NHS classes in my area were not shifting in their old-fashioned approach to educate first-time couples.'

Tamara x

This chat with Jack reminded me of why I do what I do, why I am writing this book and to never give up on promoting the importance of great antenatal education.

If you do choose to attend other antenatal education in conjunction with your hypnobirthing course, then please go in with an open mind knowing that the teacher may not be as positive about birth as hypnobirthing teachers are. I am sure your teacher will advise you on how to deal with any negativity that may cross your path if this occurs.

What sets hypnobirthing apart from other antenatal classes is that it focuses on removing fears, along with providing the tools to remain calm, relaxed and in control so that better birth outcomes can be achieved, both physically and emotionally.

We are living in times when anxiety and mental health issues are rising and this must be acknowledged. Hypnobirthing techniques are not only for birth; they are invaluable tools for life and you will be able to continue to use them after your baby has been born.

Hypnobirthing will be your best investment during this pregnancy

Let me ask you a question. If you were to be given a book for free would you value it just as much as one that you had purchased yourself? As a rule of thumb we simply don't put as much value on things that are given to us for free. I used to give away my knowledge for free when I first started teaching, in the hope of attracting more customers, but I was overlooking a crucial part of how people view money.

When my business first started doing well (and this was in the days when most people had never even heard of hypnobirthing), my friends would say to me, 'Tamara, can you teach me a course for free?' And I always said yes. My classes were always full, but I was running a course anyway so another bum on a seat didn't really cost me any extra.

I have always helped others for free without expecting anything in return. As a nurse this happened all the time, 'What do you think it might be and can you recommend something for it?' I never minded sharing my knowledge but when it came to friends attending my classes for free I would always track their progress and compare their commitment to my paying couples. Can you guess whether they practised what I had taught them with as much enthusiasm as the others in the class, or not?

The answer is of course not, and that's because people value what they pay for. Hypnobirthing requires practice and any good teacher will reinforce the importance of this as they follow your progression from class to class. Good teachers are worth paying for and you definitely cannot put a price on a positive birth experience. I must have said that over a million times in my life!

When you become pregnant, particularly for the first time, there will be a considerable amount of material products on your to-buy list. I must stress that your antenatal education should be just as high up on your list of priorities as investing in things like the pushchair because, after all, you will only get one chance at birthing your baby; the pushchair you can always return to the shop if it doesn't work out. My question to you is which is more important? The pushchair or the education to help you achieve the right birth on the day?

The ripple effect of birth trauma

This is a subject that is extremely close to my heart having been on the end of it with the birth of my son. Birth trauma can range from women being disappointed, let down or sad, to women being extremely psychologically affected. Some women swear that they will never ever have another baby let alone ever walk through the doors of a hospital again. Some women are even diagnosed as having post-traumatic stress disorder.

Sadly today we are hearing more and more cases of women suffering like this. Research and technology have made birth safer in many cases but the psychological safety of women is often overlooked. Trauma comes in many different forms; it can be an event where something happens to you or when something happens that you didn't expect.

For a woman birthing in a hospital much of this trauma can come from feeling bullied or coerced into things you didn't want to have happen. I have heard of women being forcibly examined for example, receiving interventions they really didn't want, or even someone looking down on them, raising their eyebrows or shaking their heads. Women are being made to feel extremely vulnerable in a situation where they are already vulnerable.

'I will never forget that feeling of waking up all alone, without my baby by my side let alone in my arms. My husband was upstairs in the special care baby unit at the time and I remember thinking, "Why don't I feel anything? I should feel something. Why am I not feeling like I want to see my baby right now?" I felt numb and lifeless like every bit of life had been sucked out of me. There were a lot of drugs clouding my mental state; for Serg it was the pure fear of losing us both. We should never underestimate what a birth partner has to go through when birth is traumatic.'

The ripple effect can carry on for many years. By the time I recovered from the effects of Frankie's birth it was too late to save my marriage, the emotional damage had been done. Serg has still never spoken about the trauma he experienced that day. We separated when Alana was 2 and Frankie 7 and even though it was the most difficult time in my life, it has been really interesting to witness Serg blossom into the most fantastic and loving father that I could have asked for, and for that I am so grateful. I wasn't sure whether to share with you the details of my marriage breakdown as of course not all marriages break up because of birth trauma, but in doing so I wanted to emphasize how devastating the effects can be. I learnt so many valuable lessons from Frankie's birth experience and I definitely wouldn't be writing this book today if I hadn't experienced what I did. On a lighter note I also wouldn't have met my wonderful partner Robin and gained his 2 bonus children either if my path hadn't taken this direction.

It is likely that you would have never met the midwife that will be attending your birth before, and it is for this reason that some couples look into hiring a doula to ensure they receive continuity of care along the way. This is why I hired a doula for Alana's birth and it was one of the best decisions I have ever made.

When my doula arrived at the hospital, I remember thinking to myself that everything was going to be okay. The feeling of safety and knowing I was in amazing hands gave me the confidence to birth my baby easily only a few hours later.'

Tamara x

What can be done about this?

A lot can be done to ensure that you receive the continuity of midwifery care and in an ideal world that would be a definite solution. Continuity of care means seeing the same midwife for all appointments throughout your pregnancy journey as well as having one of them attending your birth on the day. Imagine if the same midwife that you established a relationship with was then able to visit you afterwards to provide you with postnatal care; someone you can rely on who is familiar to you and someone you can trust.

Women who are fortunate to have received the ideal care such as this come away from their birth experience feeling more satisfied, with a better understanding of how and why their birth unfolded as it did, even when interventions may have been needed.

What is the result of birth trauma?

The ripples that happen from birth trauma flow into families, into motherhood, into marriage breakdowns. Children are being parented by mothers who are feeling lost and sad. The devastating events of trauma result in mothers taking little or no interest in their children, not talking to their children, not reading to their children, which of course is necessary for their language and speech development.

Trauma can cause anxiety, depression, withdrawal and physical and mental health problems. The ripple effect is enormous and if we care about society as a whole we must first care about each and every mother. Your hypnobirthing teacher may be the one to offer you this continuity of care throughout this special time in your life, as many that teach are also midwives and doulas who are passionate about supporting you throughout your entire journey into motherhood.

Chapter 4:

Education Is Your First Step

It is likely that the thoughts and opinions you currently have around birth are present because of what you have learnt about birth up to this point and this may be very limited if you are a first-time mum because you may have never thought about what it's like to have a baby until now. If you've had a baby before then it's likely you have been guided towards The Birth Path because you are looking to have a different experience this time, and it makes me so happy to know that you have found it. You are now on the right track with hypnobirthing.

When you understand how your brain works you will be able to more easily understand why you think the way you do and learn how to manage your thoughts and if necessary change them. If you do not learn how to manage your thoughts or understand how your mind works, you will not be able to make the changes that are required to remove and change any of those negative thoughts and limiting beliefs that may be getting in the way of your confidence and happiness right now. Here is an exercise to help you discover where you are right now in your head.

Exercise

Write down five words describing birth and be completely honest with your responses. You may also wish to ask your birth partner to join in with this exercise and you can then compare your responses with each other.

1 ....

2 ....

3 ....

4 ....

5 ....

The purpose of this exercise is to gauge where you are with your thoughts right now. If I was to now ask what one word would you use to describe how you are feeling about birth, what one word would you use?

I am feeling .... about my baby's birth.

Now if you were to give this particular feeling a number between 1 and 10 (1 being a mild feeling and 10 being a very intense feeling) what number would you say?

The number I would use when describing the intensity of this feeling would be …………

And lastly how would you prefer to be feeling right now about the up-and-coming birth of your baby?

I would prefer to be feeling …………………….................... about my baby's birth.

(Please revisit these same questions after you have completed your hypnobirthing course).

Hypnobirthing will teach you simple techniques to help you explore and manage any negative thoughts and feelings that you might be experiencing now whilst you prepare for parenthood. I have spent a lot of time reminiscing about where my own thoughts about birth have come from over the years, and by doing so it has really helped me to realise that the beliefs I once held were not actually mine. I had been influenced by the many people who had crossed my path over the years.

Hypnobirthing will help you to understand and explore what's going on in your head so that you can find a place of better acceptance and peace. It is necessary to remove any negative thoughts so that you don't take them into the birthing room with you when your special day arrives.

'My earliest memory of childbirth comes from my sister, Rochelle, who is 13 months older than me. We are chalk and cheese in nature even though we had the same upbringing. She was always getting herself into trouble, but when she came home pregnant at the age of 15 we were all extremely shocked. Finding out 12 months later that she was pregnant again, and then again, and again and then again was

a shock each and every time. My sister had birthed five babies by the time she was 21 years old and I was there to witness the after-effects of every single birth. What this means is that from an early age she would come home from the hospital and share all the gory details with me and she made birthing sound scary… really scary! I remember asking my sister what it actually felt like to give birth and never in a million years would I have expected the answer she gave me. Let's just say there was an image of a watermelon involved. I thought long and hard about whether to even share this with you, as the last thing I would ever want to do is add to any negative images you may already have. Let me just say for the record here and now that birthing a baby feels nothing like birthing a watermelon, but of course I didn't really know that until it was my time to birth.

Prior to becoming pregnant aged 29, whenever the subject of childbirth came up in conversation the first thing that entered my head was that horrible watermelon image my sister shared with me. I am a very visual person which probably doesn't help when I hear comments like this. Before birthing my babies this is exactly what I believed it was going to feel like for me. I'm pretty sure my sister didn't mean to emotionally scar me in this way and I wish I could have found her interpretation funny instead, but I didn't. I know this affected me a lot because when I think back to that moment now, I remember it so clearly. It's interesting, don't you think, that whenever you are in a situation that makes you feel a powerful emotion, whether that be positive or negative, it then becomes a vivid memory for years to come. This is how your opinions and beliefs are shaped and formed. It's no wonder I thought childbirth was going to be so painfully scary.

Can you think of something a parent or family member may have said to you that you still clearly remember now? If you're nodding yes then it's because whatever they said made you feel a strong emotion at the time. The interesting thing here is that my sister doesn't even remember our conversation let alone remember sharing her unhelpful and sensationalised analogy with me.

My sister's interpretation of childbirth stayed with me right up until the time I gave birth to Frankie many years later, because I totally believed that this is what it was going to feel like for me, for all women in fact! This early conditioning definitely contributed to my anxiety throughout my first pregnancy, as well as the poor antenatal education I received at the time. I now know that this anxiety could have been prevented if I had learnt ways to cope and change the negative thoughts and images that my mind was constantly focusing on as soon as I found out I was pregnant.

From epidurals to inductions, my sister had experienced birth in all sorts of ways. The births of my nieces and nephews definitely shaped my thoughts and beliefs. It made me dread the moment when it was time for me to start my own family. It's no wonder I waited until I was almost 30 to have my first child; I believe he actually chose me because my pregnancy was unplanned.

It took me a good few months to get my head around the fact that I was going to have a baby but by my first scan at 12 weeks pregnant I was very much on board with it all. I deliberately tried hard not to think about the birth at all because every time I did I would feel the anxiety creep in.'

Tamara x

When you acknowledge your negative thoughts (and by the way we all get them!) and what you can do to limit and even change them, you will feel less stressed during your pregnancy and, most importantly, less scared as you prepare for your baby's birth. You are pregnant and there is one thing for sure: your baby will need to come out at some point in the near future so you had better face this head on and stop burying your head in the sand. You will be giving birth, that is a fact, and the sooner you start preparing the sooner you will start to feel better about everything, that I do know. That was me getting tough with you! The right preparation is the key to feeling confident, and that is what you will start to feel as you embark on your hypnobirthing journey.

It doesn't matter what stage of your pregnancy you are currently at, you can start hypnobirthing at any point in your pregnancy. Starting sooner rather than later, however, is preferred so that you can more quickly gain this invaluable knowledge and start implementing it into your life as soon as possible. If you're reading this and you are quite late into your pregnancy, like I was when I found this knowledge, then now is the time to live and breathe hypnobirthing.

The importance of practice

Think back to a time in your life when you had to learn something new… riding a bike is a good example because you may remember feeling nervous and anxious in the beginning, but you persisted and worked hard at mastering the required balance to stay upright and then suddenly you were off! You practised and practised and this increased your confidence to the point where you can now just jump on a bike without even thinking about it and know what to do.

The hypnobirthing techniques will do just that. With practice they will start to feel so natural to you that you won't even have to think about what to do when applying them as they will simply feel normal and natural to you. As long as you practise of course!

If you do not ride a bike then have a think about something else you have learnt in the past, that you worked hard to master and that now comes so naturally to you it just feels like it is a part of you. This is the process of how all new knowledge is learnt. Another example is way back when you were learning to walk. You didn't give up, you just kept going and going until you mastered it and I am sure you had lots of positive reinforcement to achieve those first steps, didn't you?

The same goes for the hypnobirthing techniques. With practice they will become a normal part of your daily routine, and if you have a supportive partner around you as well then this can make a real difference to the time it can take to change any of your negative thoughts, beliefs and feelings.

How to learn effectively

Thanks to neuroscience, there is now a better understanding of how we learn and the most effective ways our brains process and hold on to new information.

I have a few top tips to help you embrace your newly found hypnobirthing knowledge.

To help with your learning, skip the laptop and take notes the old-fashioned way, with pen and paper, because research shows that if you take notes by hand you will actually learn more. The reason for this is that the act of writing out the information fosters comprehension and retention. Reframing the information in your own words helps you retain the information longer, meaning you'll more easily remember it and therefore apply it on the day when you need to.

When it comes to practising what you have learnt, only do it for a small amount of time, that way you will stay motivated to keep practising so that it doesn't become a chore. Saying that, you will be learning how to relax effectively so I'm not sure if this could ever be called a chore.

There is a strong connection between sleep and learning. It seems that getting some shut-eye is an important element in bolstering how our brains remember new information. Any mum-to-be who both practises and gets plenty of sleep not only functions better, they're also happier and so are their babies.

There are five steps to improving your concentration:

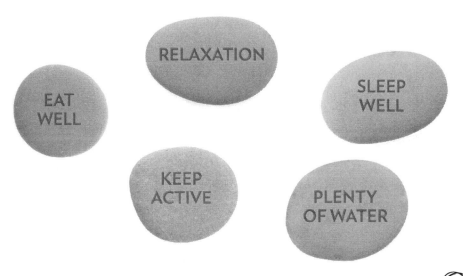

Information overload is a real thing

In order to learn something new, our brains must send signals to our sensory receptors to save the new information, but stress and overload will prevent your brain from effectively processing and storing information.

When we are confused, anxious or feeling overwhelmed, our brains effectively shut down. You might remember this feeling at school during a long, boring lesson where you may have zoned out and stopped paying attention. However, if this happens in your hypnobirthing class simply enjoy the feeling; this is a wonderful state of hypnosis and exactly what you are looking to achieve.

Drinking water is vital: it's good for your skin and your immune system, and it keeps your body functioning optimally. But staying hydrated is also key to your cognitive abilities. Drinking water can help with focus, attention and learning. Dehydration, on the other hand, can seriously affect your mental function. If you don't drink enough water, your brain will have to work harder than usual.

When you use multiple ways to learn something, you'll use more regions of the brain to store information about that subject. Your hypnobirthing teacher will cater for all learning types in class, the visual, auditory and kinaesthetic learners. Your teacher will use different media to stimulate different parts of your brain too, such as reading notes, using props, watching videos and reading scripts to you. The more resources your teacher uses in class, the more effective your learning will be.

The more you can relate a particular story to certain subjects, the easier it is to understand and grasp the point your teacher is wanting to make. I am sure your teacher will have some truly inspiring stories to share with you in class. I personally find it much easier learning something if it is connected to a story in some way. There is a point in my class where I talk about dilation of the cervix and I use the example of a birth I once attended.

'First-time mum Rachel was 1cm dilated when I arrived at the hospital. She was strapped to a monitor and sitting on the bed when I got there. With some gentle persuasion the

midwife agreed to remove the straps so that she could visit the bathroom, where we stayed for an hour with myself sitting on a birthing ball by her side speaking softly to her, with the lights off of course.

When the midwife returned she requested that Rachel go back onto the monitor, and lo and behold she started to bear down. Her baby boy was born 20 minutes later. I love this story because it shows that dilation of the cervix is often just a number and it also shows that it is possible to go from 1cm to 10cm in only an hour. A great story and a great way to make the very important point that every woman is different and all women should be treated as individuals.'

Tamara x

By the time you have finished your hypnobirthing course you will have learnt how to switch off your negative thoughts and switch on the positive ones that will better serve you and your baby at this precious time. To help you think in a more positive way you will start your journey exploring the B.R.A.I.N. Path with me. Once you have travelled this path you will then be ready to move on to the next path and then the next as you move down towards completion of all four necessary paths, and that is when you will start to feel the transformation happening.

Imagine an unopened rosebud in a garden, waiting patiently for the perfect weather to arrive so that it can finally blossom into the beautiful rose that it is destined to become. With patience, commitment and focus you too will blossom into a happy and confident parent when you experience the wisdom and education contained within *The Birth Path*. It may sound too good to be true right now and I get that, as it wasn't until I gained this knowledge, implemented it and had my daughter Alana in my arms that I truly believed and appreciated the power of this life-changing education. I am just so glad you have found it before you meet your baby too!

It is now time to start your journey...

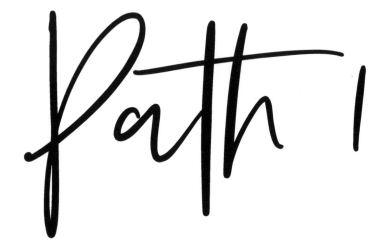

Path 1

The B.R.A.I.N. Path

The B.R.A.I.N. Path

If you truly want to remove your fear you must first be willing to change your mind!

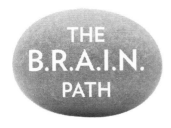

Beliefs, Reflection, Attention, Individuals, News

The **B.R.A.I.N.** Path is understanding how your brain works and why it thinks the way it does in relation to birth. I'm not talking about the physiology of the brain here. I am referring to the invisible part, your incredible mind! It's the part of the brain that is responsible for all your thoughts and feelings.

This is the first part of your journey and it is very much the area that needs the most attention when it comes to your preparation. After all, the brain is responsible for all sensations, intellect and nervous activity. It's where you register pain.

Focusing on positive themes like nature and flowers can have many benefits on the human body. Think about the emotions you may have experienced the last time you received a bunch of flowers. I bet they put an instant smile on your face! There have been scientific studies done that prove that flowers have a positive effect on the brain, they elevate mood, reduce stress and even help people to heal faster through colour and smell.

The beauty of a flower is its uniqueness! Flowers sure do make you smile and smiling is associated with positive emotions and making changes within your brain so, unless you have any allergies, why not surround yourself with plenty of flowers throughout your pregnancy as I am sure it will help you feel more positive too.

Now that I have shared the background of my hypnobirthing knowledge and experience with you, it is important that you now feel the wisdom and knowledge contained within this book will give you the confidence to go on and achieve an amazing hypnobirth for yourself. What you are about to read and learn may quite possibly be the best investment of your time and money during this pregnancy. In fact I know it will be! You have finally arrived at the beginning of the Birth Path and there is no better place to start than at the top as you discover and explore what is going on in your head right now. Let's begin by looking at your beliefs.

Chapter 5:

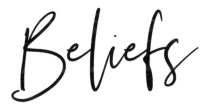

Only grow thoughts in your brain that you wouldn't mind putting in a vase

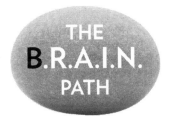

B – Beliefs

Where have your BELIEFS surrounding childbirth come from? When you REFLECT on your thoughts, memories and beliefs it affects the way you feel. What you put your ATTENTION and focus on is what you are more likely to attract into your life. The INDIVIDUALS you choose to be around can affect the way you feel and think. The NEWS and media can also affect the way you feel and think at this special time in your life.

The 'B' in the B.R.A.I.N. Path looks at your BELIEFS. If you don't explore where your beliefs surrounding birth have come from you will be unable to change them and free yourself from the detrimental effects of thinking a certain way, and feelings such as stress, fear and anxiety. If your beliefs around childbirth are negative then you will need to learn how to change them because you will not want these beliefs and thoughts affecting the way you birth your baby on the day.

When you do learn how to change your limiting beliefs around birth, you and your baby will have a much better opportunity to experience the birth that you really want and deserve.

'I remember thinking that my only choice was to book a C-section when I found out I was pregnant the second time round because I truly believed another traumatic birth was on the cards if I had attempted any other way. It was finding the right teacher and the right education that completely changed my mindset and beliefs towards childbirth, enabling me to achieve the birth of my dreams.'

Tamara x

Your belief system is the invisible force behind your behaviour. Together with other factors such as your personality, your genetic makeup and your habits, your belief system is one of the strongest forces that affects any decision you make. Your reactions to certain situations are directly related to your beliefs which are most certainly the product of what has happened to you throughout your life.

I have always wondered whether nature or nurture was the cause of my laid-back mothering approach; not a lot fazes me and I can assure you Frankie has tried and tested me many times. Like that time when he mixed every liquid he could get his little hands on in the house, including ketchup and toothpaste, to create what he called his magic potion. I am sure you can imagine the mess I witnessed when I stumbled across this in his bedroom. I can see how many parents would have reacted angrily in this situation. However, just like my own mother, I thought he was just being a creative genius and praised him for being so innovative. The question here is: was my behaviour learnt behaviour or did it come from my mother and the laid-back environment she brought me up in? I do find this subject fascinating. Have you taken on any of your parents' parenting ways? It's ok if you don't want to admit it.

You will accumulate thousands of beliefs throughout your lifetime, about all aspects of life. You will gain them through things that other people say, things you hear out and about, things you read, or any other external influences that you are exposed to. All of your beliefs are interacting with one another, affecting one another, and together form your belief system.

If you currently believe birth to be a horrendous ordeal then hypnobirthing will expose you to a different viewpoint. You are unlikely to experience instant change as this takes time, and it is for this reason that doing a hypnobirthing course with a great teacher to monitor the change and progress makes this chosen method of birthing much more effective. It will take time and regular practice of your hypnobirthing techniques to change your belief system.

If, over time, you are exposed to thoughts, information, images and beliefs that are in contradiction to your belief system, then there is a chance that eventually you will start to question some of your existing beliefs. That is the goal of any hypnobirthing teacher and what a rewarding feeling it is when we witness this shift in mindset.

Have you ever used a bottle as a candlestick holder? This process is more like wax dripping on glass constantly. It can be a slow process until you have completely transformed the look of the bottle. Eventually, the wax will be able to change the shape of the bottle, but it will take time. It is for this very reason that when it comes to implementing everything your teacher shares with you, listen carefully and diligently put into practice everything that she says, particularly how to breathe alongside regularly listening to your relaxation tracks.

Sometimes, though, we are thrown into a radically different environment i.e. a hypnobirthing class that exposes you to a completely different way of thinking so suddenly and with so much force that this process can happen very quickly. I know that some of the videos that your teacher will show you in class can have this effect. It may be difficult for you to believe that it is possible for some women to birth with a smile on their face but seeing is believing!

In my career as an antenatal educator I have witnessed many anxious mums change their minds from originally planning to have an epidural or an elective C-section for no reason apart from their intense fear of birthing, to planning on birthing in the comfort of their own homes. This is the true power of hypnobirthing and the knowledge contained within. I am not suggesting that you go out and book a home birth unless of course you want to as this is down to personal choice, but I wanted to point out how a once-held belief can be completely transformed in only a few weeks/months when you look at changing the way you view birth.

I have supported many amazing families over the years and I feel blessed to have been there to witness these most incredible transformations. I have taught many couples who have had previous traumatic births and for me this has always been the most rewarding part of the work that I do. There is nothing more incredible than finding out that a couple had a truly healing experience after such a negative one. I have always found that many of these women go on to become passionate hypnobirthing teachers themselves afterwards also.

I shared with you where my beliefs around childbirth came from before having children and you may have experienced something similar, but these beliefs can be changed and it's vital that they are. At this point you may not even realise where your beliefs have come from – and that's okay.

Hypnobirthing will help you explore these beliefs so that you can become aware of them and make the changes that are necessary to move forward without being held back by any negative beliefs. Understanding your feelings surrounding birth, and looking back into your past at why you feel the way you do about birth, is the starting point in the exploration of your beliefs surrounding childbirth.

What do I believe a positive birth to be?

When considering what is important for you with regards to your baby's birth it is important to remember that you and your midwife will need to work together. They are there to advise on the health and safety of you and your baby at all times. If concerns have been raised by your medical provider it is important to discuss these with them and find out as much as you can so that you are able to make an informed decision for yourself and your baby.

I have often been asked the following two questions:

'Are you not setting women up for disappointment by focusing on a calm, comfortable birth experience?'

'Shouldn't you be helping women by managing their expectations in case something goes wrong?'

So I thought it was important to explain what I believe a positive birth is and what it isn't. A positive birth isn't about having a short, calm, comfortable natural labour and birth free of intervention (although of course many hypnobirthing mums achieve this). It is about empowerment. Couples taking control of their birth experience, having the confidence to ask appropriate questions and making decisions, based on the answers, that are right for them, not anyone else.

So, what is my interpretation of a positive birth?

• A positive birth is the birth that is right for mum and baby on the day.

• A positive birth is one where the couple looks back and knows that all decisions were theirs.

• A positive birth is one in which mum and her birthing partner felt they were always in control, even if that meant making the decision to hand over to the experts because there were special circumstances.

- A positive birth is when a woman feels that she has had a positive birth experience no matter what path her birthing takes. I don't always get 100% feedback that birth played out in the way that was desired, but I do get 100% feedback that the techniques are useful no matter what, and that is the true value of using hypnobirthing techniques to prepare for the birth of your baby. How can that be setting a woman up for disappointment?

Always remember: Your beliefs are an integral part of what makes you think the way you do. If those thoughts are of a negative nature then hypnobirthing will help to create new beliefs that will make you feel much more confident and positive about birthing your baby.

Chapter 6:

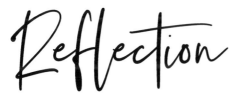

Your thoughts become lighter when you remove the negative images associated with them

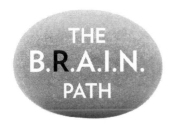

R – Reflection

This leads me into the second part of The B.R.A.I.N. Path and that is REFLECTION. Take a few minutes now and reflect. I want you to think about where your thoughts around childbirth have come from? What stories have you heard and what images have you seen? You could have feelings associated with a previous birth of your own. Maybe friends and family have influenced your thinking or even movies you've seen?

Stop, pause and have a little think before reading on…

Your response will give you a pretty good idea of how you perceive birth to be. Without exploring in greater depth why you have decided to describe birth in this way you will be unable to move forward and make any changes that are necessary to build your confidence and change your mindset. If you found positive images in your mind to describe childbirth then good for you… you might want to think about why you chose them. It's very normal to have chosen images of a negative nature at this point in time, and being completely honest with yourself right now is necessary in order to move forward towards the change you want to see.

Great! Now that you have a starting point it's time to see how we can change those images in your mind so that they can become much more positive. If you have found stories or images that portray birth as a calm, beautiful, joyous experience then that is fantastic, and shows that you are already on the right track.

I would often have midwives, doctors and other health professionals come to my classes and I would find that professionals such as these would need the most work when it comes to understanding where their beliefs have come from because, let's face it, their job is to help people who need help. When they reflect on birth they can't help but think about their job and what they have been recently faced with. If they are constantly finding themselves in situations where things go wrong then this can shape their attitude and beliefs about what they perceive birth to be.

The more you surround yourself with negative images, the more they will affect you in a negative way thus shaping your own beliefs. Some antenatal teachers find it daunting teaching medical professionals such as doctors and midwives because they are perceived as being the experts in their field (and that is often true).

We are fortunate to have them there if needed and many lives have been saved because of them. What these people aren't experts in is mindset, breathing, confidence and relaxation to ensure that both a woman's mental health and physical health are ready to give birth in harmony. Personally, I love teaching medical professionals because I know that they need this knowledge more than anyone, and have the capacity to share it far and wide.

Have a look at what one of my clients wrote when I asked him to reflect and write down his words describing birth. He has been an obstetrician now for over 10 years… I do like a challenge!!

'Monitor, forceps, haemorrhage, c-section, sutures.'

At the end of my hypnobirthing course, four weeks later, I asked him how he felt and these were the words he used to describe his baby's birth.

'Calm, relaxed, natural, choice, informed.'

There is no denying the power of great education. Wow! What a transformation in attitude and mindset. Witnessing these transformations is the most incredible part of my job as a teacher.

Tamara x

As you can see in this example above, self-reflection can help you to build emotional self-awareness. By taking the time to ask yourself the important questions, you gain a better understanding of your emotions, strengths, weaknesses and what drives you to refer to childbirth in the way that you currently do.

Reflection helps you to acknowledge how negative or positive the thoughts you have are. Acknowledgement is always the first step to understanding yourself better. There will be time spent in your hypnobirthing class to reflect on your thoughts, acknowledge them, change them and release them. This is one of the main focuses in hypnobirthing and your teacher will help you do this with an emotional fear release session in class.

Once you have understood how powerful reflection is in terms of how it makes you feel, you will be encouraged to naturally exchange any negative memories for the more positive ones. Once you have started your hypnobirthing course you will be able to more easily reflect and focus on positive images of childbirth. Your teacher will show you some truly remarkable images and share inspiring stories with you in order for you to be able to do this more easily.

You will get yourself to a place where if you are to think about childbirth, only positive images and thoughts will come to the forefront of your mind and, by doing so, leave the negative behind. This will take time particularly if the negative images you have relate to a previous birth experience, but with implementation and practice of your hypnobirthing techniques you will be able to acknowledge the effects of reflection.

In my experience, one of the most enjoyable parts of being a hypnobirthing teacher is meeting up with couples afterwards, and no, it's not just for the baby cuddles… newborn babies smell sooo good! It is a time to reflect on the birth and reframe any aspects of the birth that need exploring further, particularly for your own peace of mind. Perception is an interesting factor here and should never be taken lightly. What is important to one person may not necessarily be important to another and hypnobirthing teachers are mindful of this.

'I remember one new mum sharing with me afterwards how she really didn't like the perfume that her midwife was wearing on the day and it kept bothering her. She didn't voice her concerns outwardly but she couldn't stop thinking about it. She voiced that this was a massive problem for her during her labour and I am sure it was, but when we explored and reframed this she herself came to the conclusion that because the perfume gave her a redirected focus it in fact helped her because it served as a distraction from what was going on within her body at the time. I am sure when she shares her story with others now, that perfume is highlighted in a very different way, a more positive way.'

Tamara x

Reframing is a technique used to help create a different way of looking at a situation by changing its meaning and in this case it was decided that the horrible perfume became a blessing in disguise. It is true that even the most trivial of things can really affect your thoughts in labour which then of course can affect the way you feel.

Listening to or debriefing with clients is a significant role of any hypnobirthing teacher and I strongly advise that you contact and share your birth story with them after your birth, especially if it doesn't go to plan. Your hypnobirthing teacher will help you to reframe any parts of your birth experience in a way that can help you understand and feel better about certain aspects. This doesn't mean sugar-coating any parts where you may have felt there was a lack of care. It simply means supporting you to recognise how you used the hypnobirthing tools well in challenging circumstances. If it is beyond your teacher's realm of expertise then she will advise or signpost you to someone who can help.

Not only is reflecting on where your thoughts have come from in relation to birth important, it is also interesting to look at the much bigger picture and understand the trends behind why society as a whole views birth the way it does. In fact, our Royal Family have often set birthing trends.[4] Let's reflect on how these royal figures chose to prepare for birth.

Queen Victoria

Compared with many of her predecessors, Queen Victoria's path to multiple motherhood was smooth sailing: nine pregnancies all carried to term. Victoria nonetheless appreciated the burden of birth, and when she heard about a method of pain relief, she grasped it: anaesthesia.

In 1847, the Edinburgh obstetrician James Simpson demonstrated that chloroform could dull the pain of childbirth so she demanded it.

---

4 https://www.historyextra.com/period/victorian/royal-baby-family-women-childbirth-birth-labour-labor-history-meghan-markle-victoria-mothers-traditions/

Simpson anesthetised the queen by dripping chloroform onto a handkerchief stuffed into a funnel through which she breathed. 'The effect,' wrote Victoria in her diary, 'was soothing, quieting and delightful beyond measure.' Queen Victoria used anaesthetic again for her final delivery, Beatrice. This chosen birth method required birthing in a hospital rather than at home, thus setting this trend for many to birth this way.

Queen Elizabeth II

When Princess Elizabeth, the future queen, was ready to give birth to her first child in 1948, it took place in the Buhl Room at Buckingham Palace, normally a guest room with a lovely view down The Mall.

Who was in attendance at this home birth? Not Prince Philip. He played squash during Charles's birth, bringing champagne and carnations to Elizabeth after it was over. But he did attend the birth of his fourth child, Prince Edward, in 1964 – as have all royal fathers since.

The Duke and Duchess of Cambridge

We have all been waiting with baited breath for Catherine, Duchess of Cambridge, to reveal the details of how she birthed her babies. Many newspapers and magazines reported on Kate's hypnobirthing preparations with much speculation, but finally, in February 2020, Kate shared her experiences with the world. In a live interview on the *Happy Mum Happy Baby* podcast with another hypnobirthing mum, Giovanna Fletcher, she spoke about how beneficial the hypnobirthing knowledge and tools had been for coping with morning sickness and all three births.

Kate said: 'I saw the power of it really, the meditation and the deep breathing and things like that – that they teach you in hypnobirthing – when I was really sick and actually I realised that this was something I could take control of, I suppose, during labour.' She continued: 'It was hugely powerful and, because it had been so bad during pregnancy, I actually really quite liked labour!'

The Duke and Duchess of Sussex

Harry and Meghan are the latest couple whose pregnancy and birth choices have attracted much interest. They took a personal decision to keep the plans around the arrival of their baby private. It has been reported however that Meghan and Harry looked into hypnobirthing and a doula for the birth of Archie, but this has yet to be confirmed by the couple directly. After much speculation around a planned home birth it was later confirmed that baby Archie was born in a London hospital.

The media's interest, reporting on hypnobirthing being connected to both Kate Middleton and Meghan Markle, has definitely encouraged more couples to look into it as an option which can only be a positive and progressive way forward! It was an honour to be contacted by the *Daily Mail* when the news came out; I was interviewed as the hypnobirthing expert to accompany this news in a great article that can be found online.

Self-hypnosis requires reflection

Hypnosis is a focused state of awareness that requires you to reflect on certain parts of your life as a way to make any necessary changes. Let's reflect on what hypnosis is and how it can help you.

Over the years my life has been complex and uncertain. Maybe yours has been as well? But I've learnt to make more effective choices in my life, and using hypnobirthing techniques has allowed me to achieve a more relaxed and calmer sense of living. The hypnobirthing method focuses on teaching you how to become an expert in relaxation and your hypnobirthing teacher will show you how to do this.

As hypnobirthing uses self-hypnosis, a good place to start would be to define what hypnosis is and what it is not by dispelling a few myths for you.

Often people's first experience of hypnosis is by either hearing about or seeing a stage hypnosis show. I thought, therefore, that it would be best to 'get out of the way' any preconceived ideas that this may have created. It is common to perceive hypnosis as what you might see on stage: doing silly things whilst in a state of trance. They must surely have no idea of what they are doing. Why else would they be prepared to make such fools of themselves?

However, when someone goes to a stage hypnosis show they go with one of two thoughts in mind:

• either to watch a show and to be entertained or

• to be part of that show and participate in it.

If it is the latter then there will already be a suggestion within them that they are going to be asked to do silly things. They are a willing participant. Once the show commences, the hypnotist will ask for anyone who wants to be part of the show to come up on stage. He then proceeds to use hypnosis techniques to take these people into trance whilst at the same time looking for the best candidates to work with. Those he feels are least likely to respond to his suggestions will be asked to leave the stage until he is left with the few he believes will provide the most entertainment.

When the hypnotist brings a person out of trance and asks if they believe they have been hypnotised they will most likely say no. This is because there is no particular 'feeling' of being hypnotised. However, on reflection when they talk about their experience they will say it felt similar to a time when they had a bit too much to drink. You know you could stop yourself saying or doing something, you may even know that you should, but the alcohol gives you an excuse – it quietens the more rational side of the brain. I have often heard people say it just feels like they can't be bothered.

Often the most suggestible people for a stage hypnotist to work with are those who want to be more gregarious, and perhaps you see them 'coming out of their shell' after a few drinks. It is important to note, however, that even if the hypnotist has been appearing to get individuals to do the most ridiculous things, if he asked something of them that went completely against their moral code such as 'What is the pin number to your bank account?' they would not respond as this is something that you would never want to share with anyone.

The subconscious (i.e. the parts of the brain that we have no conscious control over – more on that later) does not make moral judgements, so your conscious brain can cut in at any time, and the person would either just ignore the suggestion or open their eyes and come out of trance. Whether a stage hypnotist, a hypnotherapist or your hypnobirthing teacher are working with trance, they are actually utilising a natural state that you go in and out of every day.

Every time you give your focused attention to something, be it a good movie, a book or staring into the eyes of the person you love, you are in a state of trance. When you are daydreaming about something, drifting off to sleep or just waking up, you are in a state of trance. You are not fully alert nor are you asleep since you are aware of things around you, and yet you are giving all of your attention to your own inner thoughts and feelings.

When we are fully conscious and aware, we have a critical factor of the brain that acts as a filter. This filter has been established in accordance with our belief system and is what we use to analyse incoming information. When we move into a state of trance this becomes side-tracked and we therefore become more open to suggestions. This is important to be aware of, because both positive and negative suggestions can get through.

There is a lot of negative hypnosis about childbirth. Every time you hear a horror story you are drawn in by the imagery that it creates, the critical factor of your mind is momentarily side-tracked and the negative suggestion that childbirth is awful is planted. If this happens enough times it will become part of your conditioning. When used therapeutically, and how we use it in hypnobirthing, trance is a very good state for changing outdated beliefs and absorbing new learning.

A useful side effect of entering into trance in this way is that you also access what is known as the relaxation response and this produces a state that helps counteract the negative effects of stress on the body. So, simply being in this state is highly beneficial and, in particular for birthing, being in a deep state of relaxation is the key.

What does it feel like to be hypnotised?

Often, hypnosis is described as an extremely relaxed state. Certainly, that is what you will be aiming to achieve when using hypnobirthing, but it is not always the case. I have shown below a number of different natural states of trance and you will see that some promote relaxation and others most definitely do not. In fact, during a formal hypnosis session we all experience trance in a different way. Some people feel very heavy as if they are sinking into the surface on which they are resting, others feel light and tingly as if they are beginning to float, and some feel nothing at all but are just aware of the voice they are listening to or their own inner thoughts.

There will be times during a session when your mind may drift off, whilst at other times you may become more aware. The most important thing is not to try: the more you try the more you will engage your conscious brain and will be less likely to move into the state of trance. You should simply set the intention to allow yourself to experience trance in a way that is just right for you. Instead of judging how you feel, know that it is working for you in the way that is best for you. Some feel different and some do not, and so you must focus on what you are hearing and not what you are feeling.

Trance will then happen all by itself. Let's take a look at some natural states of trance and you will find that one of them occurs when we are watching a 'good' movie. I think this illustrates trance brilliantly. I want you for a moment to think back to the last time you were at the cinema watching a thriller or a horror movie. You are so caught up in the imagery that you let go of reality for a while and, whilst watching, you believe what you are seeing to such an extent that you actually feel the suspense, the anxiety and so on.

At the same time however you still have an awareness that you are in the cinema. That awareness is greatly reduced but it is still there and in fact if it wasn't, that would be horrific for you as you would genuinely believe that the film you are watching is real.

When you experience trance during a hypnobirthing class it is nice to know that there is a part of you that remains in control as this is what gives you the confidence to consciously let go and get the most from the session. Let's look a bit closer now at some other natural states of trance. You will see from this that you go in and out of trance many times quite naturally, so there can be no doubt in your mind whether or not you can be hypnotised.

Daydreaming

Daydreaming is something that occurs naturally any time the subconscious feels it needs to remove us from our present surroundings (mentally not physically of course). This can be because we are bored, unhappy, or just have a lot on our mind. Wherever our mind wanders off to at that moment, we believe we are there.

Storytelling

By an individual or through a film/TV etc.

When we get caught up in a good story we temporarily let go of reality. We no longer give attention to where we are but get transported to the experiences of those we are hearing about or watching. Although it is not our reality our body will physically respond to what we are experiencing all the same. We cry at extreme sadness, we feel frightened at a scary scene, we jump at a loud noise and so on. It is not physically happening to us, but in the moment we are reacting as if it were real.

Fixation

Have you ever found yourself just staring off into the distance, perhaps staring into a fire or looking up at the clouds floating by in the sky or maybe even just a crack in the wall? The mind has simply wandered off and is no longer fully present, enjoying the peace that this brings.

Driving

For those who drive a car I bet there have been times when you arrive home after a familiar journey and wonder how you got there? Physically active and yet in a complete state of trance. The subconscious has already been programmed for home and with the suggestion to take you there, it does it all by itself.

Shock

When something completely out of the ordinary occurs most people don't know how to react as they have no frame of reference to tell them how to respond. They have moved into a state of trance and become highly suggestible. They will then follow the instructions of anyone who takes charge. We will explore this in more detail later when we look at avoiding unnecessary intervention.

Emotions

Any highly emotional state will place us in a state of trance. It is easy to spot how we become less rational when we are scared, angry or sad. How we perhaps become more suggestible when we are highly excited with a group of friends having fun. If you ever see a couple in a restaurant newly in love you will notice that they are completely oblivious to those around them; they are in the zone, blocking out the rest of the world and focusing, feeling and connecting purely on each other in the moment.

Sex

For most of you this is what has brought you here in the first place. Even for those who needed some assistance in getting pregnant, you still had the same driving force that led you to wanting a baby in the first place. Sex is one of the best examples of trance – assuming you are enjoying it of course. You get completely lost in what you are feeling, letting go of any thoughts or cares of the day or even where you are. It is also a great example of overriding the critical factor of the brain; your partner perhaps can say a word that appears completely innocent to anyone else yet to you the suggestion has been made. You get the picture – you don't need me to explain any further.

The above are all great examples of hypnosis and as you can see some will support a relaxed state but others most obviously do not.

Suggestibility

When we have been formally hypnotised we become much more suggestible but, as we have seen from the above examples, we can also be very suggestible during naturally occurring states of trance. Anything that draws us in emotionally, positively or negatively, will have the ability to bypass the critical factor of the brain and make us more open to suggestion. The level of success these suggestions will have will depend on:

• the importance we may give to the information in the first place

• who is delivering the message

• how the suggestion is given.

It is important to be aware that your mind is already working in this way. Everything you will be learning, your mind is doing already. You will just be looking at things in a slightly different way in order to make sure that your mind is working for you and not against you.

Myths

A section on hypnosis wouldn't be complete without looking at the myths surrounding it.

Getting stuck in hypnosis

This can no more happen than a person getting stuck in sleep or a daydream. If an individual doesn't come out of trance it is because they are enjoying themselves too much. A person trained in using hypnosis with people will know how to respond appropriately to this. If you drift off whilst listening to one of your hypnobirthing tracks and you don't come back with the count you will either drift off into a nice relaxing sleep, coming back when you are ready, or when something more important grabs your attention.

Hypnosis is harmful

Hypnobirthing scripts are written with a focus on building confidence for a positive birth experience. That said, when you enter into formal hypnosis, your conscious mind will maintain some presence, however slight, and therefore your moral values and ethics will never be overridden. The only hypnosis that is harmful is the naturally occurring trance we may go into on receiving negative information.

Understanding your mind and its connection with your body

Understanding how your mind is working and the impact it has on your body will enable you to get the very best out of the techniques that you will learn in your hypnobirthing course.

The human mind can be split into two quite different parts: the conscious and the subconscious. We use the conscious mind for all our intellectual thinking. It is rational, critical, analytical and judgemental and with its short-term memory it can only focus on the 'here and now'. It is also responsible for the voluntary actions of our muscles and therefore has some control over our nervous system.

The subconscious mind represents over 80% of your brain's capacity and is responsible for our creativity and imagination. It has a huge memory store containing the 'learnings' acquired from all the experiences we've ever had, including every piece of knowledge and skills we've gained and any associated emotional responses. The subconscious mind also controls the autonomic nervous system and the immune system and therefore looks after all the functions of the body that we don't have to consciously think about, for example our heart beating, our breathing, the functioning of our uterus, etc.

We make decisions and take action using the current information gathered by the conscious mind combined with the 'learnings' stored within the subconscious mind. Once a decision has been made, the conscious mind then constantly reassesses the situation to ensure that the correct action has been taken, using the same evaluation of current and past information. It is often believed that the conscious part of our mind is the strongest. However, because the conscious mind cannot make any of its decisions without first referring to the 'learnings' stored within the subconscious mind, we can clearly see that the driving force behind our actions is indeed the subconscious. The understanding of this is vital to our success when we want to make a change.

Many people attempt to make change using the conscious act of willpower; some are successful but most are not. Their lack of success is caused by the subconscious continually trying to pull them back to what they know. You may well ask, if the conscious mind has rationally understood that change is necessary, why would the subconscious mind sabotage its attempt at change? The answer to this question comes back again to survival.

The primary role of the subconscious is in fact our survival and therefore the only thing it really cares about is whether we are safe or whether we are in danger. When we at first attempt to make change it believes we are placing ourselves right in the middle of a danger zone. I know this may still not be making sense yet, but stick with me.

In a deep state of relaxation (hypnotic state) there is no difference between real and imagined

The subconscious mind doesn't understand words but responds to the world through imagery.

It runs your body – all those things that happen without you thinking about it (heart rate, salivation, perspiration, breathing rate) – by using emotional responses activated by that imagery.

Because it responds to the world through imagery and emotion it doesn't know the difference between real and imagined events. Think about watching and hearing someone scratch their nails down a blackboard. How does that make you feel? Argh!!! Because it uses imagery and the associated emotional responses to run your body, it will make changes in your body based on what it perceives as your reality (whether those changes are actually needed or not).

Because its primary role is our survival, once it has learned something it then looks for other things that are similar so that it doesn't have to spend precious time working out what is dangerous and what is not for each and every thing we come across. Let's look at how the subconscious was functioning back in prehistoric times. The needs of men and women during prehistoric times were simple to understand.

They needed shelter and protection (both from the elements and other animals), warmth and food to survive and companionship in order to reproduce. If any of these needs were not met it would generate a fear response to stimulate them into taking the necessary action. Without these things they were in fact in DANGER. Once all of their needs were met they felt satisfied and SAFE.

It was very clear to the subconscious what it needed to do. When it had to activate the body for action and when it could relax. Now let's look at what the subconscious is up against in modern day, developed countries. Our needs now are not so simple to understand. Luckily for most, the prehistoric human's needs are no longer an issue (certainly not in any way to such extremes), but there are many things that make us feel stressed, anxious and even afraid that are not about our immediate survival. However, because the subconscious is responding to the emotion, it is setting up the body for danger all the same. It believes that we are in physical danger.

If something has been causing us to feel this way for a long period of time the subconscious learns to protect us from whatever that is. It has in fact learnt incorrectly that this 'thing' is a threat to us. When we try to tell the subconscious simply through willpower that it learnt its lesson wrong, it doesn't want to listen because it believes that it has been keeping us safe. Let's look at an example of something we quite rightly are afraid of. Coming face to face with a snake! We know some snakes are dangerous.

Imagine that a snake charmer has just walked into the room with a snake and informs you that it is the friendliest snake you will ever come across and you can stick your hand in its mouth. Would you go straight up to that snake and do just that? Probably not! Some will do it more quickly than others, some will need a lot of convincing and some will never put their hand in its mouth. Even if you did, you wouldn't then stick your hand into any old snake's mouth as you know some of them can be poisonous. Your subconscious has learned correctly that some snakes are dangerous. This is an important fact for you to have learned for your survival. Simply being told that this particular snake won't hurt you, will not be enough for most to accept without further reassurance and emotional preparation (if you have a phobia of snakes or anything else then hypnosis can help).

How do the messages get learnt?

As we grow and develop from a very young age we hear messages from those around us about what is safe, what is not, what is right, what is wrong, etc. This evokes a corresponding emotion, which in its most simplistic form will equate to a feeling of either safety or danger. If we hear the same message enough times this is what we believe. At a young age we don't have the mental ability to question this, so everything we learn is accepted as fact.

During prehistoric times this was a simple process, but now there are so many variables that it can be very easy for us to learn things that are not necessarily useful and even inappropriate. In fact, every time we hear a negative story about birth and it makes us feel frightened we are further reinforcing the message that birth is a difficult event. Unfortunately, the subconscious translates that to 'birth is a dangerous event'. Birth without special circumstances is not a dangerous event and therefore the lesson has been learned incorrectly.

We may also learn something that some have considered useful for us at one point in our life, but as we grow we realise that this is no longer the case. We may consciously start to realise this but the subconscious is still under the false illusion that it is keeping us safe. It is here that we need to make the change. I wonder how many reading this were subjected to a horrific example of childbirth during their sex education class as a teenager? I think some misguided teachers believed this would prevent young girls from having sex and getting pregnant but sadly the most likely thing it achieved is a woman frightened of giving birth. Consciously, we can learn something new and useful but the subconscious will inadvertently be sabotaging our attempts at success. In order to make changes at a subconscious level we must do two things:

1   Change the emotional attachment to the past. More about that soon.

2   Repeat new ways of thinking in order to change our habits of thinking. As mentioned previously we learn mainly through repetition, and when we want to change the way we think this is actually no different to when we want to learn a new skill.

How we learn new information

We can understand this further by looking at how you learnt to drive a car or ride a bike. Let's use driving a car as an example.

There is a time when we are very young that we don't know what driving is and are therefore unaware of a lack of skill. At some point we realise that the vehicle we are moving in involves someone having to manoeuvre it and the idea of driving becomes known to us.

When we are ready to learn the skill of driving we take lessons, but we are very much consciously driving – having to concentrate on the different things we need to do in order to be able to drive competently. Once we have passed our test and gain more experience we do not notice so much about every detail of our driving; we are responding automatically to what is happening around us, even singing along to the radio or chatting with a friend. Then one day we arrived home and cannot even remember how we got there. On the one hand fully active and responding appropriately, on the other in a complete state of trance.

Think back to how you learnt to ride a bike; you were conscious and aware of everything that was going on around you and really focused on mastering the required balance. Once the training wheels (stabilisers) were off you were then able to enjoy the normal and natural feeling of riding a bike, like it was a part of you, and you then let go of thinking about it all so much.

You will find the techniques that hypnobirthing teaches you will feel just like this too. At first they may seem strange and require much of your focus but with practice you will find that they become second nature. It simply takes time, practice and patience.

Let's look at a lesson that your subconscious may have learned incorrectly, that you want to change

The message that birth is a difficult experience, something that many women dread.

Before finding out about this birthing method you may have felt frightened in some way about birth, believing that it is something that you will need to endure in order to have your baby.

You found out that some women had no such fears, and in fact were excited about experiencing birth, but you don't know how that could be possible.

You attend a hypnobirthing course and learn what caused you to have such fear, along with a set of tools to help you change the way you feel.

With practice of these tools and listening to the hypnosis sessions regularly you find that it has become second nature for you to think positively about birth and simply feel excited about meeting your baby. Often when we start to feel uncomfortable with the status quo, out of sync, or just have that feeling that something isn't right, it means you haven't quite learnt all that you need to know. We may not have even realised that we had been picking up information that was suggesting our current way of thinking wasn't working for us, but the moment we realise this is the point at which we need to take action, which means looking for ways to make change at a subconscious level.

Conscious desire for change

The subconscious doesn't like change. So, during the initial period of time needed to reassure it that it actually just learnt the lesson wrong in the first place, you must have a clear idea of why the change is so important. Changing the way you think is necessary; it is no good learning a whole new set of facts about birth and then still focusing on all the horror stories. Whatever we think about drives our actions and, therefore, if we consciously focus on a positive birth experience, we will be more driven to practise the skills we are learning. If we focus on the negatives we might wonder 'what's the point?'. We call this a conscious desire for change. Do not underestimate the importance of this. If you do not tap into this conscious desire for change your current subconscious programming will override your attempts for change and you will not have the driving force to put what you will learn into practice. Know now that you deserve a positive birth for you and your baby. Focus on what you want, not on what you don't want, and tap into that desire anytime your subconscious tries to pull you back to your old ways of thinking and behaving. The more you practise your hypnobirthing techniques and listen to your hypnobirthing tracks the easier it will become, until one day you find that you have reached a place where the techniques you have been putting into practice have simply become a new way of thinking.

Your brain has been trained in a particular way over time.

Let's see how you get on with this very simple exercise. How many letter 'F's can you count in the following sentence after reading it only once?

FINISHED FILES ARE THE RESULT OF YEARS OF SCIENTIFIC

REFLECTION AND STUDY COMBINED WITH THE EXPERIENCE OF YEARS.

How many did you find? Now read it again. Did the number change? Maybe you counted only three or four when in fact there are a total of seven 'F's in this sentence. If you found seven straight away then well done you; I'm not sure it means anything apart from this exercise didn't work for you. Why not see how this works for your partner?

If this exercise worked for you then you will find that your mind did not register consciously what you read. You would have read the word 'of' as 'ov' which is why it is likely that you skipped those particular words. It's a great exercise. When I do this in class most people only find three or four but it doesn't have anything to do with IQ. It is simply how we have trained our brains over time to read in a certain way; and of course if you can do this you can train it to do other things too like focusing on birth in a positive way anytime birth thoughts float your way.

Always remember: Hypnobirthing will enable you to reflect on any birth images or birth memories that come to mind in a much more positive way so much so that you and your birth partner will start to look forward to your birthing day.

Chapter 7:

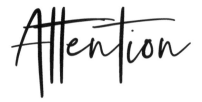

To bring positivity and confidence into your life, imagine that it's already there!

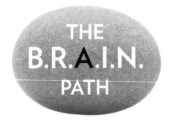

A – Attention

The third part of the B.R.A.I.N. Path is 'A' for ATTENTION. I like to call this the 'think it to feel it' stepping stone. This is all about shifting your focus so that it works for you by making you feel better. When you think about it and then feel it you will receive it. Are you ready to give yourself permission to feel good? You may have heard about 'The Law of Attraction' or in other words what you focus on is what you get! If this is your first time hearing this then you might want to do some further research on this topic. There is, in fact, a lot of science behind the principle, also known as quantum physics if you are a more evidence-based person in nature.

An easy way to describe 'The Law of Attraction', and in fact the way that I describe it to my children, is to imagine that you are a walking magnet. What you feel and focus on is what you will attract into your life. Now without sounding too woo-woo here, what if what I am talking about is true and if focusing on a certain outcome makes it more likely to happen? Why wouldn't you?

Would you not agree that by doing so it really wouldn't take up too much of your time either? So, whether you believe in this way of thinking or not, how about just for now and just while you are pregnant, you make a conscious effort to focus on the birth that you want to have and avoid thinking about the one you don't want to have. After all, there really is no point rehearsing a negative one.

In my hypnobirthing classes I ask couples to focus on their birth like it's already happened.

'I did what you said and I wrote an email to you at 30 weeks pregnant pretending that my baby had already come. It went like this:

Hi Tamara, I wanted to share my amazing news with you. My labour started gradually which was great because it helped me get used to the surges. I easily breathed through them right up to the point when I felt pressure down below. When I arrived at the hospital I was greeted by a warm and caring midwife who knew all about hypnobirthing. She was so happy to see how calm I was. I remember the amazing feeling I got after getting into the pool and lucky I did because 20 minutes later my baby was born. It was the most amazing feeling of my life and I feel so proud to send you this email.' Heather, first-time mum, London

Heather's actual birth was pretty similar to what she wrote in her message above, apart from the time it took her to birth once getting into the pool. It was two hours not 20 minutes; however once time distortion kicked in she describes it as feeling like it only took 20 minutes (time distortion is another positive effect of hypnobirthing and it simply means that time can feel a lot less than what it actually is).

If you don't learn how to change your focus and attention while pregnant not only can this increase your anxiety levels, but also the confidence you will need in order to move forward and prepare for your baby's birth with a stress-free approach. Let's face it, life is so fast and busy these days that I am sure you can do without any extra stress.

When you learn how to focus your attention in a way that is beneficial for you and your baby you will naturally build your confidence and start to really look forward to your special day, and that is what you and your baby deserve. The techniques that you will learn in your hypnobirthing course will enable you to give attention to the areas in your life that will serve you best.

'I am not a visual person so instead of focusing completely on what would be my perfect birth, I realised throughout the classes that my perfect birth is one where I feel in control and confident in myself rather than the environment that I was in. I would imagine myself feeling calm and in control rather than what the scene looked like. This has helped me make birth plans that I'm really happy with and am looking forward to my labour rather than thinking of it as an unpleasant means to an end.' Lindsay, second-time mum, Dubai

Imagine now that you are a painter, creating pictures of your life and then making choices and taking actions related to your masterpieces. What if you don't like the picture? That's simple, change it! Your life is a blank canvas of possibility and you are in control of what that finished picture could look like. Once your picture is finished think of it often and make it yours to have.

You could even get creative and make yourself a 'birth vision picture'

To help you attract the birth that you want, why not create a 'birth vision picture' (also known as a dream board) and place it somewhere in your house where you are likely to view it often. If 'The Law of Attraction' is something that resonates with you this exercise can help turn your dreams into a reality.

The main purpose of a birth vision picture is to help you examine your desires and empower you to focus on what you really want to happen during your baby's birth. To assist in finding the appropriate images that are meaningful to you, why not start with an image of your relaxing place in nature as this is where you will visit in your mind throughout labour. Then select images that represent your birth desires. This will help you to narrow down your focus and personalise your board with choices that matter to you. For example, you might want to add an image of a birthing pool if you have decided on a water birth. It is thought that the process of making these choices sends a very specific and personalised message to your subconscious mind and the universe about your desires.

Visualisation is nearly as powerful as performing the action and your brain trains your body to prepare for action. When you imagine yourself stepping into a birthing pool, for example, your brain runs through the process and sends signals to the rest of your body to complete the action. When you visualise yourself in the birthing environment that you want, your brain trains your body for the reality. Every time you repeat this visualisation you will become stronger with that action.

Creating a birth vision picture and placing it in an area of your house so that you can see it often will ensure that you are creating the opportunity for you to visualise consistently so that you will be training your mind and body to manifest what you truly want for your baby's birth. The wonderful thing about a birth vision picture is that it only requires your time and energy for the initial creation. After that the consistency in the visualisation happens every time you stare at it. It can also influence the thoughts of anyone else around you so that they too can focus in a positive way.

For more information on the 'The Law of Attraction' visit:
www.thelawofattraction.com

Birth affirmations

'I put my attention on my chosen birth path. I concentrate all my efforts and energy on what I most want to accomplish for the birth of my baby. I focus on what I most want to achieve.'

Tamara x

Birth affirmations are an integral part of any hypnobirthing programme. They are positive statements written in the present tense to help you practise new ways of thinking about birth. They help get the conscious mind in sync with the aim of a positive birth experience and give an alternative to any negative thinking.

Affirmations are a structured way to practise new thoughts and at first it will be useful to set a time each day to focus on these. In time, positive thoughts about birthing will become your new habits of thinking and give you the best opportunity to have the birth you seek.

These are available for you to listen to, but you may also like to read them, or copy some down and place them around your house or in your workplace, so that you can spend as much time as possible focusing on your calm, comfortable, relaxed labour and birth. The more you listen to them the more you will start to believe what they are saying to be true, thus changing your attitude to a more positive view of birth and way of thinking.

Here are three of my favourites. Why not make up some of your own so that they are specific to what you want to focus on and achieve?

- 'I am relaxed and really looking forward to the birth of my baby.'

- 'I approach the birth of my baby feeling calm and confident.'

- 'I feel calm, relaxed and in control during labour and my muscles work together in complete harmony.'

Tamara x

Your affirmation exercise – Write, record, revise, repeat

It is likely that your hypnobirthing teacher will give you a recording to listen to throughout your practise, however if you would like to tailor-make your own personal birth affirmations here's how:

- Write down your personal affirmations. Use language such as 'I am,' 'my baby,' 'I feel' etc. Be mindful of your language and, of course, be as positive as you possibly can.

- Record yourself (or your partner) on your mobile phone.

- Repeat each affirmation twice (add some relaxing music in the background if you wish).

- Listen consciously and repeat out loud the repeated affirmation (obviously this depends on where you are and who is around).

You may have noticed up until this point that I have put a lot of my attention on sharing why I think you need to do hypnobirthing. Here are the steps you can take to make sure from this point onwards that your attention is focused on the best possible birth that you can achieve. Here are the three most important steps to take on your pregnancy journey so please pay attention.

The necessary steps

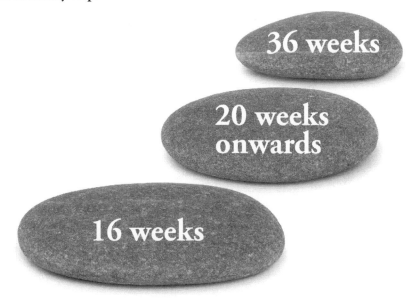

- 16 weeks – Start researching your hypnobirthing teacher.

- 20 weeks onwards – Book your hypnobirthing course.

- 36 weeks – Practice, practice, practice all techniques.

Always remember: Hypnobirthing will help you attract the birth that is just right for you and your baby. We call this the 'right birth on the day'.

Chapter 8:

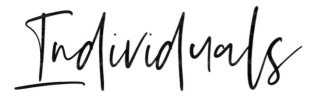

Comments and words affect you only as much as you let them!

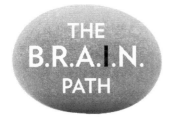

I – Individuals

It is really important to understand how other INDIVIDUALS can affect how you feel whilst pregnant as it seems like it is human nature to share negative birth stories with others without even thinking about how damaging this can be for you. In the fourth part of the B.R.A.I.N. Path we look at how you can be easily influenced by other people whether they be friends, family, work colleagues or even the medical professionals that you are having your check-up appointments with.

I am sure you are nodding your head right now and thinking back to the last person who shared their opinions with you. I have always wondered why so many people, particularly women, feel the urge to share a negative birth story with you just as soon as they find out you are pregnant. Why do they do this and do they really think they are helping you?

This really does puzzle me and maybe it's because I am slightly removed from the reality of this as I make it a practice to not share negativity about birth because I know how much it can influence people. I am not saying negative things don't happen, of course they do, but why would you give your attention to something that has nothing to do with you. It is after all their story, not yours!

At the beginning of this book I mentioned how I deliberately don't share with others the details of my traumatic birth because I do not want to add to any of the negative images that may be going around your head right now. You don't need to know why my birth was so traumatic but you do need to know what I did to make sure it didn't happen again. I was very much influenced by the antenatal teachers that crossed my path each time and I have learnt that not all teachers are experts in their chosen field even if they say they are.

When I booked my antenatal classes I didn't even question what my teacher Beverly was teaching me, even though a lot of the information was shocking and she focused on all the things that could go wrong. I believed her and as a first-time mum, I was hanging onto every word she said. I just didn't know that birth could be another way. A lot of what she taught me also reaffirmed what my sister had experienced which, of course, reinforced to me what childbirth was like. After leaving her classes I remember focusing on all the things that could go wrong; I couldn't help it, I just expected my birth experience to be painful and horrible. I will talk about the importance of expectancy, another form of hypnosis, when we explore what pain is further on down the track.

My teacher was definitely an expert in preparing me for the worst outcome, I give her that. No hypnobirthing teacher would ever do that and in fact the focus will very much be on the opposite which, of course, is everything that can go right! I believe it is important to not blame her entirely, of course, because she wasn't there with me when I went into labour, but if I could relive that time in my life I would have asked this individual a lot more questions and I am sure my husband would have too.

If you prepare for your baby's birth without considering the influence of individuals around you, the negative suggestions that they can plant in your head can have a detrimental effect on the way you feel whilst pregnant and the outcome of your birth experience. Your hypnobirthing teacher will teach you how to avoid any negative influence from others and how to protect yourself from the effects of this on you and your baby.

The impact of others

It is a sad fact that the general population hears more horror stories of birth than good ones. We can forget this as we tend to hear only positive ones, but unfortunately in the main, women continue to be brainwashed into believing that birth is a difficult and traumatic experience. This is something that is passed down from generation to generation and amongst peers, and as each woman then experiences her own difficult birth so it continues. In fact this happens so often that women who experience a positive birth say that they find it hard to share, as they are considered lucky or even that they are showing off.

The media plays its part too. Films, soap operas and birth channels all know that calm, relaxed births are not 'sensational' TV and so rarely show positive ones. Although, to watch a woman labouring calmly is the most sensational thing you could want to see. As we now know, this expectancy is a form of hypnosis. A woman who is convinced that birth is awful will only notice the negative stories. If she does hear a positive one she will dismiss it as luck.

In effect, her subconscious is filtering out anything that doesn't fit with the belief that birth is difficult. On the other hand, a woman who believes that birth can be a good experience will notice many more positive stories about birth and her subconscious will be seeking ways to further prove that what she knows is correct.

Hypnobirthing will teach you how to protect yourself from any 'glass half empty' individuals

Whenever someone shares a difficult birth story with you or you watch a dramatised birth on TV there is potential for the critical factor of your brain to be side-tracked. Whilst you are being caught up in the emotion of the story your subconscious mind becomes wide open to receiving yet more negativity about birth, thus creating more fear. When this happens your subconscious mind can then get further clarification that birth is a scary and dangerous event.

This is negative hypnosis and I urge you not to get involved in negative conversations about birth; stop people in their tracks when they want to share a horror story particularly about birth and don't be tempted by the birthing channels as their views are often one sided. You will find plenty of wonderful hypnobirths to watch on YouTube or visit The Wise Hippo Facebook page.

How ever determined you might be you will block any of the above influences, sometimes you just aren't in a position to stop someone sharing, or you might be in another antenatal class where the other couples want to hear about all the pain-relieving drugs and interventions that may take place. It isn't words that impact us but the emotions that those words evoke. For this reason it is important that you learn how to protect yourself emotionally whilst pregnant and of course your hypnobirthing techniques will help you with that. It is the emotional attachment you put on things that determines how important they are to you.

'You mean, you didn't just stop at the petrol station to get me a birthday card this morning?'

'I arrived home at 9am this morning ready to enjoy my annual birthday-card-opening ceremony. I made a coffee, got comfy and wondered which one to open first. There were cards from family in Australia, homemade cards from the kids and many others from various friends but there was one card that overshadowed

them all. The card from my good friend Nic. It just felt special, it felt thoughtful, it had deep meaning. My first thought was I wonder where she found it and when did she find it... has she been holding on to it for months waiting for the 9th of July to come? I'm sure you'll agree that words are powerful because of the emotional connection we attach to them but on this occasion it wasn't the words as such, it was the picture that spoke to me so much more. We often hear the phrase 'a picture can speak a thousand words' and in this case it did, thus the inspiration behind writing this post today. It is obvious that the person responsible for posting this card chooses things carefully and takes the time to do so... unless she just got lucky which of course is possible too. This friend didn't just go for the first or even cheapest card in her local shop. She made time to look around and really think about the message and meaning behind the card before posting it to me and that makes me feel special... well that is how I chose to perceive it anyway, even if it isn't true. Yes, but it's only a picture of a silly-looking hippo I hear you say! Well to you it might be but for me it means so much more and it's just like everything in life, isn't it? Because would you agree that it is the emotional attachment we put on things which determines how important they are to us? This friend knows I love hippos, after all my hypnobirthing programme is named after one "The Wise Hippo" but there is something about this patchwork hippo that really resonates with me today. She is a bit wonky, colourful and a bit all over the place. Sound like anyone you know? I am sure my kids will vouch for that! Patchwork; something composed of miscellaneous or incongruous parts, hodgepodge; pieces of cloth of various colours and shapes sewn together to form a covering. Well blow me down, now I know why!!!! It's all about putting the pieces together and finding the ones that fit best to create the bigger picture and an amazing end result. As a teacher, trainer, doula, this is what I do.....that hippo on the card is me!!!!. I love the metaphor here in terms of the decision-making process as it's just like the important message that I often find myself sharing to expectant couples out there. When things are important to you, like having a positive and empowering birth experience for example, it is vital that you gather as much information as you can, do your research and come up with the perfect plan on how to prepare and piece it all together for your baby's birth. Do this and you're likely to have a much better end result and of course the right birth on the day! When putting together

The Wise Hippo Birthing programme® it was important that I pieced together all the wisdom I had gathered from not only my own experiences but also from the amazing birthing women, midwives, doulas etc. that had crossed my path along the way. As I sit here and reflect on my life, my friends and family, it is clear to me that this fab card perfectly represents my patchwork life and I am sure the hippo will more than likely represent how I will be feeling after my birthday dinner and cake later on this evening.'

Tamara x

Tamara Cianfini, personal Facebook blog post, 9th July 2019

Taking responsibility for your thoughts is therefore key to your success

It is important to understand that it is only what you think that is important. If you find yourself in conversation with someone who just cannot understand that you expect your birth to be a positive experience and one that you are looking forward to, do not get drawn into a debate. This could be damaging to your self-confidence and even plant negative suggestions about your ability to have the birth you want.

Here is a useful statement that you may wish to share with those who doubt your ability to have a positive birth experience: 'I have chosen to prepare for birth using The Hypnobirthing Method, because I want to achieve the best birth possible for myself and my baby. I have learnt simple, yet powerful tools and techniques to help me remain calm, relaxed and in control, along with knowledge that I feel empowers me to make choices that are right for me and my baby on the day. By doing this I know I can have a more positive birth experience no matter what path my birthing takes.' If this person has experienced or seen another person have a very difficult birth and they do not have the desire to accept that it doesn't have to be this way, they will never be able to accept your way of thinking. For the sake of your birthing experience, accept that they have a different opinion to you and move on. If you know beforehand that someone has a very different idea of birth to you, don't even go there. If they try to share horror stories with you just respectfully say to them that you would rather wait until after you have had your baby and share stories then. Change who you listen to and you will change the way you think and feel.

How to swap your thoughts with a 'brain shuffle'

This technique is so simple to do, it's just the remembering part that needs the most practice. The 'brain shuffle' is a great way to ensure that you do not allow your negative chatterbox to take over. Negative thoughts are simply a habit of thinking and, with your conscious desire for change clear in your mind, you can easily move away from them.

Remember that because your subconscious mind responds to the world through imagery and emotion, it doesn't know the difference between real and imagined events. Therefore, irrespective of whether the way you are feeling is relevant to what is happening to you in that moment or not, your subconscious mind will believe that is your reality.

That little devil on your shoulder may be responsible for saying things to you like, 'You can't do this, you're not strong enough, you have a low pain threshold. Just because she can do it, it doesn't mean you can', and so on. Who you need to listen to more often is, of course, the little angel on your other shoulder because she makes much more sense and is much more useful when it comes to you feeling more positive. She will say to you, 'Of course you can do this. You are perfectly designed to have a baby. You have all the strength within you to do this and hypnobirthing will support you every step of the way, go girl!'

Before you continue though, it is necessary for you to understand that this is NOT about ignoring difficult feelings, or distracting yourself from important issues that need to be addressed. This is about those worry thoughts around things that are not real, for example negative thoughts about your birth experience. The 'brain shuffle' works because your mind cannot hold two opposing thoughts at the same time.

How to do the 'brain shuffle'

You may want to close your eyes to do this exercise after you have read all about it.

• Think of something that makes you feel sad or has a negative feeling associated with this thought – a person, place, food; the first thing that comes to mind.

• Now think of something that makes you feel happy and has positive feelings associated with this thought, the first thing that comes to mind is the right thought for you.

• Now think about both these thoughts, the negative and the positive at exactly the same time.

• You will quickly notice that you can't. You can switch between the two but you cannot think about them both at the same time. So, all the time you are focusing on the positive thought you can no longer focus on the negative one and from the subconscious perspective all is once again right with the world.

• You will see that you cannot have two opposing thoughts at the same time: a simple example of how your brain works and of how you have the power to decide which thought to focus on.

As soon as you find yourself focusing on a negative thought you will want to exchange it for something more positive. Because your thoughts evoke a corresponding emotion, the way you are feeling will most likely be your first indicator that your negative 'chatterbox' (the devil on your shoulder) or negative 'self-talk' is speaking to you. If the way you are feeling is not relevant to your immediate situation it is worth checking in on your thoughts. If they are those worry-type thoughts, full of 'what ifs' and 'maybes', they are most certainly not useful to you and you will want to exchange your thoughts with a simple 'brain shuffle'. It really is as easy as that!

Firstly, thank the thought for attempting to be of use to you but firmly tell it that it is not a crystal ball and therefore doesn't know what the future holds. Shake (or shuffle) your head, say the word 'NO' to yourself or out loud if you prefer, and then mentally push the negative thought away whilst pulling in the positive thought that makes you feel good.

Become aware of the imagery of that thought in a way that is best for you. Some will see a moving image, others will be more aware of the sounds that were part of the experience or perhaps the textures and feelings associated with it. Whichever way you experience it doesn't matter, just whatever is right for you and if you smile at the same time this will enhance the positive feeling.

It does take practice – your subconscious will be comfortable with what you are currently doing. But the more you make the effort to do the 'brain shuffle', the easier it will become. By doing this, you will ensure that your subconscious isn't needlessly getting you ready for an emergency state.

Instead, you are ensuring that all body functions are working normally. The 'brain shuffle' is useful for any area of your life but, of course, the focus of hypnobirthing is for you to have a positive birth experience. Therefore, use it to keep any negative thoughts about birthing in check. As soon as you become aware of anything negative about birthing, whether it is coming from you or something/someone external to you, exchange it for a positive thought that makes you feel good.

If this can be about birthing then great. However, the important thing is that you are no longer focusing on the negative and are instead feeling great whilst imagining something positive. You may find that the positive images of childbirth that your hypnobirthing teacher will share with you in class can help you find a memorable image. Below is an example of two very different thought processes. Remember you have the power to take charge of your thoughts.

'I have been mentally preparing myself for the worst-case scenario, running the negative images over and over again in my head, the silence of the sonographer

when something is wrong, the stillness of my baby, the trauma that birth will be and then the knowledge of knowing that it's likely that I will have to go through it all again.'

Or

'I have been mentally preparing myself for the best-case scenario, running positive images over and over again in my head, the smile of the sonographer during my scan, my active baby moving inside me, the joy that birth can be and the knowledge of knowing that I will enjoy this journey now, achieve the right birth on the day and then even do it all again in the future.'

Focus on the birth you want to have

An important aspect of getting what you want is focusing on what you want. In the case of your baby's birth, the first step may even just be knowing what you want. It is something we don't necessarily spend much time thinking about. We hear horror stories, we learn about physiology, we know about the different places we can birth, who may support us and so on, but we don't tend to really think about what we want to experience.

The normal response, in fact, of a first-time mum is 'How can I know what to expect when I haven't done it before?' or if a mum has had a previous difficult experience she may say she can't imagine how it can be different. What they are really saying is that they can't imagine what it will feel like; although, because of the horror stories, they may well have already 'tried' to imagine the worst pain they can to 'try' and work out how it might feel.

What they are in fact doing here is rehearsing a difficult outcome. The more they imagine pain, the more potential there is for fear and we all now know where this can lead. Because the subconscious doesn't know the difference between real and imagined events, it will make changes in the body either way. Whenever you think about the labour and birth experience you and your baby will have together, you always want to imagine the most positive outcome.

Thoughts are the means by which we shape our experiences. We know that as we think, hear or read something we create images, which in turn evoke emotion. This emotion is then used by the subconscious mind to interpret what it needs to do in order to run the body and in turn take action. It is therefore useful to spend time daydreaming about your calm, gentle birth as if it has already happened. This will evoke positive emotions, teaching your subconscious mind that birth is indeed something that can be enjoyed.

Always remember: The individuals you choose to be around whilst pregnant can affect the way you feel about your baby's birth. Always remember if an individual attempts to share a negative birth story with you, you may wish to stop them in their tracks. It is their birth story, not yours! Hypnobirthing will teach you techniques to filter out negativity and encourage you to surround yourself with positive people.

Chapter 9:

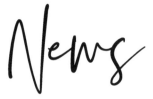

Read all about it!

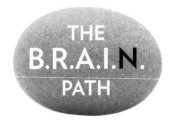

N – News

The last part of the B.R.A.I.N. Path is all about the NEWS and the media that you might be surrounding yourself with or even movies or television shows that you have watched in the past. I am sure these shows have coloured your thinking and beliefs surrounding childbirth.

You may even have noticed friends posting their news regarding their baby's birth on social media with possibly too much detail of how horrible and painful it was for them. Most publicly shared news, as I am sure you are aware, is often doom and gloom and negative in nature. We rarely see positive images of childbirth in the media unless we actively search for them and even then they are hard to find.

I once appeared on a TV show called *First Time Mum* teaching a reality TV star named Ferne McCann. Initially I thought, 'Do I or don't I?' and then I thought, just maybe, this could be a great opportunity for the media to show birth in a positive way, so I jumped at the chance. I was intrigued to learn her thoughts as I knew that she was going through an extremely stressful time in her life. My techniques and MP3s were going to be exactly what she needed. Ferne started her hypnobirthing journey by listening to The Wise Hippo morning sickness MP3s (you are welcome to download these for free in The Wise Hippo shop at www.thewisehippo.com).

I taught Ferne The Wise Hippo Birthing programme® as well as supporting her on the day. I am so very pleased to say that she achieved the right birth on the day, a beautiful natural birth. But when the programme aired the primary focus was on … can you guess? Ferne saying how painful it was during the moment of birth. What the media failed to mention was that she stayed at home during most of her labour relaxing in the bath, using the breathing techniques I had taught her and going for a lovely walk in her favourite place in nature. Ferne birthed her baby within two hours of arriving at the hospital, which is fantastic but of course this was never shared on television in this way.

Another example of the way that the media can twist the meaning of things is to take another look at England football captain Harry Kane's Instagram post pictured in the earlier part of this book. To me this post represents a proud husband feeling over the moon about achieving a wonderful hypnobirth, and rightly so. What is wrong with that? Once the media got wind of this they reported that Harry was turning birth into a competitive sport, suggesting that if some women chose to have pain relief then they had failed somewhat. How crazy is that? I just hope he remembered to use his 'Cloak of Protection' (That's a Wise Hippo technique by the way).

Even if your birth doesn't go to plan on the day, there is a lot of power in knowing and seeing that birth can be a positive experience. Your hypnobirthing teacher will enjoy sharing with you incredible birth stories as evidence that what she is teaching you, works. Seeing is believing after all!

When you do learn how to avoid the negative images in the news and media you will start to reprogramme and change the thoughts and images that are currently in your head. You will learn some really useful techniques that you can use to replace any negative images with positive ones in your hypnobirthing class.

The UK news reports that the world's first recorded hypnobirth was in 1957

A letter received by the Positive Birth Movement on 12th September 2019

'Hello, I love that you are trying to spread the idea that giving birth is an act to be enjoyed, and I thought that you might be interested in my story. I am 85 now, and 62 years ago I gave birth under hypnosis, and the whole journey was filmed for the BMA. It was an amazing experience, the film was used for some time by various groups, but I have no idea what happened to it in the end. It was reported at the time in a couple of national newspapers and it made headlines locally. I believe it was the first time that hypnosis had been used for childbirth under medical guidance.

I suppose that I was one of those fortunate individuals for whom childbirth came relatively easily, at least at first. My first child, a girl, was born quite quickly after a fairly short labour, but afterwards I had a bad attack of the Baby Blues – postnatal depression it would be called nowadays!

My doctor at that time was a friend, as well as our GP, a very forward-thinking and clever man, and he suggested hypnotherapy as an alternative to drugs to help my depression (he had begun to study the subject and I think he saw me as a possible 'guinea pig!'). So he began to take me for hypnotherapy sessions, and they proved to be very successful.

Sometime later I became pregnant again, and at this point my doctor suggested that I might consider taking part in a study of birth under hypnosis, under the BMA, as he was looking for a suitable candidate for his proposed participation. I should point out that he considered that I was suitable, given the success of our previous therapy. I believe that one of the factors that made me a good subject was the fact that I knew him very well and had complete trust in him and his judgement.

After discussing it with my husband and getting his agreement we began the sessions. The first of which were to train me to first of all completely relax, and then subsequently to be able to enter the hypnotic state listening only to the doctor's voice. This was apparently to see if the therapy would work for a group of people, rather than just a one-to-one situation. He made a tape recording of his voice leading into the state at which he could then give the directions needed to achieve a relaxed and pain-free birth.

A local journalist became interested and he invited her to sit in on one of the sessions, during which he demonstrated that I could be quite deeply in a hypnotic state and feel no pain. He had me stretch out my arm over the side of the couch, suggesting to me that it was as strong as a branch of a tree, and then proceeded to sit on it! That surprised me as well as the lady watching! He also put a couple of needles through the skin on the back of my hand and again I did not feel pain. I felt the sensation, but no pain.

On another occasion, I had dental treatment under hypnosis, not an extraction, but some quite invasive drilling! This all sounds quite dramatic, but it demonstrated the possibility to control pain, without drugs, and without taking away sensation. I think that it was really to prove that a woman could feel the sensation of childbirth without being distressed by pain.

During this time he began to prepare the introduction to the film which he could eventually make of the birth itself, well not him personally, but we had a local photographer making the film, and he arranged for the birth to be filmed at the local maternity hospital. I had my first baby at home and had planned to have this baby at home too, but the doctor said that the BMA wanted it to be shot in a hospital setting. This caused some difficulty; I wasn't booked in at the maternity unit, therefore the staff would not be attending, but we could use one of the labour rooms! In fact, I did have a midwife with me, a lovely lady gave up her off duty to help!

My due date, according to the doctor, was early July, and I began contracting on June 24th. Had I been having the baby at home I would not have thought it necessary to call the nurse or (in this case) the doctor as the contractions were about ten minutes apart or more.

However, knowing that my first labour had been short, it was a bit of a panic to get the doctor, the photographer, and all the filming equipment to the hospital on time. The labour stopped, and the midwife told me that the baby would have been quite small if I had given birth, she believed that the dates were wrong! She was proved correct, for despite the cervix being about five centimetres dilated, I finally went into labour properly on August 12th!

I later thought that as the doctor had said early July, that the implanted instruction had given me a false labour! Who knows! Anyway, I had a seven and a half pound boy! We had no access to the kind of screening available today, relying on the date of the last period and the experience of the midwife!

Well, there we were, in the hospital, in established labour, and my doctor and all the entourage were milling about getting ready for the big event, and my training kicked in nicely, I was progressing exactly as planned, well in control, and not suffering any pain. My midwife, bless her, was in attendance but as soon as they arrived, the doctor took over, giving me additional support with his hypnotherapy technique. The baby was born quickly, too quickly as it turned out, because I pushed too soon and damaged my cervix, which did give me some problems later.

There were several important lessons learned as a result of this birth from a medical point of view, and I wasn't told all of them, but one thing I do remember was that my blood pressure remained constant throughout the labour and delivery. This is apparently unusual and caused some comment from medical personnel when the film was shown.

About a month after the birth I was invited to attend the first showing, at the maternity hospital where he was born, for doctors and midwives. That was odd, as I saw the birth from the camera's angle, and did not remember some aspects! The people who saw the film were all very interested, and asked lots of questions, both of myself and my doctor! Then the film was shown to interested groups elsewhere, but I did not attend these showings.

The papers picked it up, of course, front page news for the local paper, the Essex Chronicle, for a couple of weeks, and it made the Daily Mail as well! I was invited to speak at several women's groups, and I was happy to do so, as I felt that the experience could have a very positive effect on the way childbirth was handled in the future. It is gratifying to know that now the use of hypnotherapy is being made part of prenatal care!'

Edith Barr, aged 85

What news is the Royal College of Midwives (RCM) sharing?

Physiologically the way we give birth has, of course, not changed. But many things associated with childbirth have changed, including:

- Women's expectations of childbirth.

- Pain-management options.

- The economics of childbirth and the system of healthcare.

- The technology used during pregnancy and birth.

These factors have greatly changed women's childbirth experiences.

What is the RCM?

The RCM is a charity for maintaining and improving the standards of professional midwifery. The Trust conducts and commissions research, publishes information, provides education and training and organises conferences, campaigns and other events.

The RCM says:

'England remains short of midwives, a situation openly acknowledged by the Government.

The RCM's new estimate, based on the number of births last year and the number of staff in post, is that the country's NHS is short of the equivalent of 3,500 full-time midwives.

After several years of negative trends within the midwifery workforce in England, we are starting to see some more positive trends emerge. We have a commitment from the Government to train 3,000 more midwives over and above existing plans. We are starting to see an improvement in the number of younger midwives in post, helping to address the longstanding issue of the age profile of the profession.

There has been an 80% increase of births in women in their 40s since 2001. Older women will typically require more care during their pregnancy and postnatally. This will not be true in every case, but overall it does add to the mix of complexity with which maternity services must cope. The very clear ageing of the profile of women accessing maternity care does therefore increase the number of midwives needed by the NHS.'

State of Maternity Services Report 2018 – England

The average age of mothers is now 30.2 years. This increase in the average age of mothers may be due to a number of factors such as increased participation in further education[3], increased female participation in the labour force, the increasing importance of a career, the rising opportunity costs of childbearing, labour market uncertainty, housing factors and instability of partnerships.

Office of National Statistics UK

I thought it would be extremely useful for you to gain a little more insight on where our maternity services are right now to give you a better picture of the difficulties that many women face on their pregnancy journeys. Your hypnobirthing teacher will ensure that you have all the information you need in order to wade through the many issues listed above, and if your circumstances are beyond your teacher's realms of expertise she will know how to signpost you to the appropriate information.

Always remember: The news that you hear, the books that you read, the programmes you watch, and the social media platforms you visit will all influence your thinking. You will be shown some incredible hypnobirthing footage in class that will definitely inspire and reprogram any negative images that the media may have been responsible for creating in your mind up to this point.

Path 2

The B.O.D.Y. Path

The B.O.D.Y. Path

'My goal is to fall in love with my pregnant body that will birth my baby!'

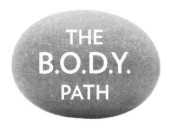

The next part of *The Birth Path* looks at your incredibly well-designed body. As a woman you have been put together in such a way that carrying and birthing a baby can happen just as nature has intended. There is, of course, a percentage of women who are unable to conceive or birth a baby due to special circumstances, but for the purposes of teaching here I am talking about the majority of women who are having a healthy and straightforward pregnancy. If you do have a special circumstance remember to consult your midwife or doctor about it for specific advice relating to the alternative paths that you can take.

I have always found it interesting that, no matter how many births I attend, the more I see, the more I learn as a teacher too. There are two main things that I have learnt on my teaching journey so far and you may want to log these in your memory bank:

• No two births are ever the same.

• There are no absolutes. What I mean by this is that anything can happen when it comes to birth and you cannot foresee how your body and baby will respond to labour on the day.

There is a vast difference between women who have educated themselves with breathing and relaxation techniques beforehand compared to women who haven't. Not learning about what your body is intending to do on the day seems futile in my opinion. When I see women birthing as nature intended, primal, focused and determined, I am completely in awe of them.

Your body is an incredible machine that can grow another human being! Have you ever just sat back and thought about how clever you and your baby are? When you can fully understand what your body needs to do on the day to get your baby out, you will be able to focus on this incredible event in a more positive way.

When you learn about the physiology of your amazing body and connect with the how and why it is built the way it is, you will be able to more easily manage the feelings that are associated with the surges and labour. Without understanding how your body works, you could more easily feel out of control and tense up when it's time to birth your baby and this can lead to a whole cascade of interventions for you and your baby. Hypnobirthing is all about exploring ways to enable your mind and body to simply do what they are perfectly designed to do.

'One of the most valuable parts of my hypnobirthing course was learning about the physiology. My surges felt like an unstoppable force of nature that I just had to accept. I knew exactly what my body was doing and why it was doing it, I would describe it as a powerful and necessary feeling that needed to happen and knowing this kept me in control throughout my labour.' – Karen, Sussex

Chapter 10:

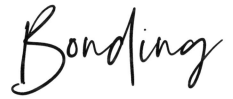

Close your eyes, connect, imagine and smile…

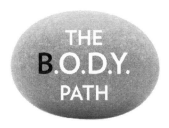

B – Bonding

It's time now to explore the 'B' in the B.O.D.Y. Path. Without knowing about the importance of this, you may go about your way without ever noticing that your baby has feelings too. What if they have been trying to communicate with you in their own special way but you have been oblivious to these messages? What I am talking about is BONDING both physically and emotionally with your precious baby.

We now have more knowledge of the importance of the prenatal period than ever before. With advances in research, medical science has now been able to provide 'proof' with increasing evidence that a baby's parents' lifestyle, emotions and external environmental factors are all important to their development. There is now no longer a place for the nature vs nurture debate, with recent findings showing that the baby's genes and its environment are actually working integrally together. Whilst your baby is growing physically they are also developing emotionally.

The unborn baby is tuned into its mother's activities, learning about the 'rhythms of life' and their associated emotional responses. An important lesson we can learn from this research in fetology teaches us that the more consideration parents give to their baby during the time in the womb, both in terms of their environment and emotional wellbeing, the more likely their child will be able to reach their full potential. It is important to be aware of your feelings and emotions during pregnancy because your emotions will affect the way your baby behaves and feels.

For example, when you are upset your baby's heart rate will rise and when you are feeling happy your baby will get an extra burst of endorphins and feel happy too. With this in mind, you can look for ways to create the best environment for your baby; but also bear in mind that part of our emotional learning includes some of the more difficult emotions too. Your children will see and experience examples of sadness, anger, frustration, etc., after they have been born and as they grow, and there may be times that it is appropriate for you to display those feelings during your pregnancy.

In fact, it is of great importance that you are able to express your feelings. You will find your new skills will be useful during those times, to help you feel emotionally in control, and by doing this you will be creating a strong foundation for your child with regards to their emotional intelligence.

Prenatal bonding exercises

Whether you are aware of it or not there is communication taking place between you and your baby. From your baby's perspective their external communication will be shown through their movements. What does your baby do when you go into a room with loud music or sit in a warm bath? You may find that they become aroused in these situations showing you that they are aware of the change in environment and that they are responding to the stimuli around them. You may wonder whether there is any point talking out loud to your baby. Research has shown that once babies are born they respond to the stories they heard whilst being carried. They really can hear and love the muffled sounds of your voice and those around you. It is common to receive feedback from mothers reporting that their babies continue to recognise their hypnobirthing music as newborns by having a calming effect on them. I have even had partners in my classes say that they have become so accustomed to listening to their hypnobirthing tracks whilst going to sleep that they can't go to sleep without them.

Did you know that it has been proven that a baby can distinguish their father's touch from an unfamiliar hand whilst stroking your tummy? So why not have your partner touch or stroke your tummy? If your baby responds with a kick, your partner may want to press back. Do this a few times and then change the pattern.

Of course you can play this game with them too, as can any siblings or other family members and close friends. Friends and family playing with the baby before they are even born! Your practice together will teach the baby that when your birth partner speaks or strokes you, be it daddy and/or someone else close to you, that you relax deeply.

When the baby is here they will respond to their voice and touch in the same way. This is the same for mum too. Talking, singing lullabies or telling a story whilst you are feeling relaxed and calm can condition your baby to respond and be soothed by those things after they have been born. Quite often we instinctively start to talk to our babies without even knowing it and we are right in doing so. Communicate with your baby in any way that feels right for you, knowing that not only is this enhancing your baby's development but your baby is having fun communicating with you too. If you haven't already chosen a name for your baby, you may like to give your baby a 'pet' name, instead of referring to your baby as 'it'.

'Call me super sensitive but something that felt really important to me whilst pregnant was to protect my bump as much as I could from technology and what I mean by that is not holding my mobile phone or any other electronic devices near my baby bump. I would keep my phone in my bag rather than my pocket too. I'm not sure why, it just instinctively felt like the right thing to do. It also meant that I had more time to focus on my baby rather than being constantly distracted by phone calls and social media. I even made up a personal affirmation for myself, "I unplug to connect!"'

Tamara x

Your baby's ideal position for birth

Your baby is connected to you in the same way as all other parts of your body. The mind/body connection can influence your baby's position too. What you imagine can make changes in your body and therefore you can influence your baby's position by imagining them in the ideal position for birth.

It was my doula and hypnobirthing teacher Suzanne who shared this wisdom with me. I remember her showing me a picture of a baby in an optimum birthing position with the words underneath that read: 'head down, chin to chest, hands to heart and back to belly.'

These words became my mantra and I would close my eyes and imagine my baby in this position every day of my pregnancy.

How can being more aware of your emotions help you to connect with your baby?

Hypnobirthing helps you to understand your emotions and behaviours associated with them. Becoming more aware of how your emotions make you feel is the first step towards looking at ways to become more positive about birthing your baby. For example, if you're feeling happy you may decide tonight is the night to sit down with your partner and chat about birth planning, but

head down
chin to chest

hands to heart
back to belly

if you'd been let down by a previous birth experience then the decision to do this might trigger all sorts of emotions again such as fear and disappointment, so you decide to avoid this conversation and find something else to talk about instead.

This is a simple example of how your emotions can control your behaviour. Another example might be if you have had a water birth before or you know of another person who shared their water birth story with you, then those details will be what you reference when thinking about water birth. Isn't it interesting how your emotions can be a direct response to something that you may not have experienced personally? I am very much hoping that the emotional state that you will experience after reading this book will be excitement and that you will take action and find yourself a great hypnobirthing teacher to support you.

Birthing your baby will be one of the most emotional times in your life. Without hypnobirthing techniques in your back pocket and if a negative emotion were to surface, such as anger or frustration, you might end up making decisions hastily without considering the implications. If you feel afraid, your decisions may be clouded by uncertainty and caution, which can affect the decision-making process. Hypnobirthing teaches you and your birth partner to trust your instincts as well as paying attention to the way you are feeling. Hypnobirthing will help you:

• Change any negative moods and attitudes.

• Quickly manage any stress and anxiety.

• Stay connected to what you feel as well as think.

• Follow through on your hopes and dreams.

As you develop the capacity to better recognise and understand your own emotions, you'll find it easier to appreciate how your partner is feeling too. Maybe it's your partner who is feeling anxious and you are looking at hypnobirthing as a way to help them feel more positive? It may be the case that this baby has come along unexpectedly (both of mine did!) bringing up all sorts of emotions that you haven't experienced before (mine was definitely a shock. Both times!).

As you learn how to bring stress into balance and learn to tolerate even unpleasant emotions, you'll discover that your capacity for experiencing positive emotions will grow and intensify. This is great when it comes to bonding with your baby. You'll find it easier to play, laugh, and experience joy when thinking about their birthday, no matter how stressed or emotionally out of control you might be feeling now.

With hypnobirthing, life can and will get lighter and brighter. The shared goal of all hypnobirthing teachers is to get you to a place of feeling calm and prepared to deal with anything that crosses your path on your birthing day. The last thing you need right now is to be constantly playing out negative birth scenarios in your head.

What is rumination?

Has your head ever been filled with one single thought, or a string of thoughts that just keep repeating themselves? The process of continuously thinking about the same thoughts, which tend to be negative, is called rumination. A habit of rumination can impair your ability to think and process emotions. It may also cause you to feel isolated and can, in reality, push people away. If this sounds familiar to you then talk to your hypnobirthing teacher about which tools can be specifically helpful in this situation.

If this resonates with you and you do get stuck in a ruminating thought cycle, it can be hard to get out of it. If you do enter a cycle of such thoughts, it's important to stop them as quickly as possible to prevent them from becoming more intense. Hypnobirthing techniques are designed to help you do this quickly and easily knowing that you can have full control over how long you wish these thoughts to hang around. It's easy when you know how!

So, what can you do to stop these negative thoughts from running through your mind?

Here are some tips for you to remember in times when that same thought starts swirling around in your head:

• Remember the 'brain shuffle' technique.

• Distractions can help and the hypnobirthing breathing is a great way to take your mind off what is going on.

• Thinking more about how your troubling thought might not be accurate may help you stop ruminating because you realise the thought makes little sense.

• Setting realistic goals that you're capable of achieving can reduce the risks of overthinking your own actions.

• Think about how you can improve your self-esteem.

• Your hypnobirthing relaxation tracks are designed to increase confidence.

• Knowing how to breathe.

• Ruminating thoughts can make you feel isolated. Talking about your thoughts with a friend, partner or family member who can offer an outside perspective may help break the cycle.

• Therapy – however, hypnobirthing is a great first course of action. Your hypnobirthing teacher can signpost additional help if needed.

It's also important to be proactive and book your hypnobirthing course early, as the sooner you do the sooner you will be taking the necessary steps to prevent yourself from ruminating in the first place. With the hypnobirthing knowledge in place and some lifestyle changes, it's possible to free yourself from ruminating thoughts.

What is the rewind technique?

Something else that can be useful, particularly in cases where birth trauma has been experienced, is something called the 'three step rewind technique'. Ask your hypnobirthing teacher if this is something that she can offer you. I have used this technique many times both personally and with clients and have witnessed some truly remarkable emotional shifts. Attending a hypnobirthing course is a great start to combat the effects of any birth trauma and I am sure your hypnobirthing teacher will recommend any further help if it is necessary.

Your heart-felt focus session

It is now time to get creative and really connect with your emotions. The following exercise will take you around 20–30 minutes to complete. It's a great way to explore your emotions and if you do it together with your birth partner you may find that issues come up that can create some really useful discussions for both of you. You may discover that your partner is worrying about certain things that you have been completely unaware of. This exercise is a great way to lay it all out on the table before your hypnobirthing preparation begins.

You will no doubt be feeling mixed emotions as you focus on your baby's arrival and with that can come some difficult feelings too, causing you to feel not so good. Please know that these feelings are simply there to relay a particular message to you. This practical exercise will help you and your partner explore what those messages are.

Practical exercise *(drawing stick figures is of course most welcome in this book!)*

Part One: Connect and Create

- You will need paper and a pen/pencil for this exercise.

- What are you worrying about in your life right now? This is about exploring what message there is for you in your emotions.

- Spend a few minutes now focusing on what emotions you are currently experiencing by turning them into images.

- Connect with your emotions and create the images that are causing you to feel this way, e.g. Worried about putting on weight? Scared about next scan? Confused about home birth vs hospital birth? Money issues? Draw it.

Part Two: Feel and Reflect

- Write down your feeling/feelings against the image/images you have drawn, e.g. how does this image make you feel when you look at it?

- What is the message behind this emotion? Write a brief explanation about how you are currently responding to the image you have drawn. What is this emotion making you do/not do?

- You may or may not wish to share and compare your images with your partner at this point. Have you found out that your partner is worrying about something you were unaware of? The emotions you are experiencing are real to you even if those around you aren't experiencing the same.

Part Three: Change and Create

- Now revisit your images. How can you redraw or adapt it in any way so that your feelings associated with it become more positive? Go ahead now and redraw the image/images. (It may be the case that you now draw the opposite to what you have already drawn.)

- This simple exercise will ensure that you are truly responding to the message of your emotions. This works in a similar way to the 'brain shuffle' that you learnt about earlier.

- Changing the visual images associated with the emotion you are experiencing can be a really useful and healthy habit to get into.

Now that you have become more aware of your emotions you can revisit this exercise throughout your pregnancy to ensure that you are acknowledging your emotions so that you can handle them in the best way for you and those around you, including your baby.

Play your favourite tunes and boogie with your baby

Dancing is an excellent way of keeping you healthy, flexible and stress-free during your pregnancy. You don't have to be a great dancer to enjoy the benefits of dancing with your baby. What music makes you want to get up and dance? Your baby will love the feeling they get when they feel you moving and enjoying yourself so why not start each day with a little boogie, or better still end your day dancing around the living room to your favourite tunes? It's a great way to celebrate pregnancy, keep fit and connect both physically and emotionally with your baby.

• Dancing can increase your flexibility, fitness and muscle tone.

• It's a great alternative to the gym.

• Helps with blood circulation by keeping your heart and lungs healthy during pregnancy.

• Dancing will increase your energy levels and uplift your emotional state.

Always remember: Hypnobirthing will encourage you and your birth partner to connect inwardly with your baby so that you can nurture them both physically and emotionally during this special time in your life. Being aware of your emotions and how they can affect your baby even before they are born is so very important for you to understand.

Chapter 11:

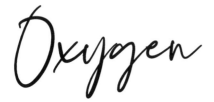

You and your baby need oxygen. You have so much in common already!

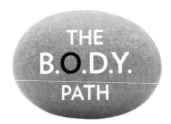

O – Oxygen

The vital ingredient for survival and life. I am sure you know that without OXYGEN you would not be able to live and if your oxygen supply was reduced you wouldn't be able to function effectively either. Now, to keep this birth-related you need to understand the importance of this chemical element and how it can affect your body and baby in labour.

When you understand why your body needs the right amount of oxygen and how to ensure you do all you can to effectively oxygenate your body during labour, your body and baby will then be able to work together in harmony during labour and birth.

Breathing correctly in labour will help with your oxygen supply. When your breathing is shallow, which happens when you are scared, you are not getting the amount of oxygen that your body needs. Your blood needs this oxygen because it is the blood within your body that will supply your uterus muscle with the necessary oxygen it needs to function efficiently. A lack of oxygen in your blood can affect the way your uterus contracts making your surges weaker and less effective, making labour longer.

'I remember arriving at a birth and noticing how shallow and fast her breath was. She reported that her surges had stopped and she looked worried. I asked her to close her eyes and focus on my voice as I guided her gently back to the breathing techniques I had taught her so that she could calm down and increase her oxygen supply. Then, in no time at all, her surges started again and she went on to have a beautiful birth only four hours later.'

Tamara x

Your oxygen supply, in addition to breathing correctly, will be the key to you staying in control and being able to manage your labour on the day. Your hypnobirthing breathing techniques will be the most important of all. The slow and controlled breathing that you will need to master before your labour begins will make all the difference to the way your body responds on the day.

'Another memory I have is of a conversation I once had with a midwife who shared with me what the uterus muscle looked like in a frightened woman she was caring for in theatre. As her Caesarean birth was underway she could see the colour of the woman's uterus and it was almost white. What this meant was there was hardly any oxygenated blood supplying the muscle. Failure to progress was the reason why a Caesarean birth was recommended on this occasion (She was not a hypnobirthing mum).'

Tamara x

Calm and relaxed breathing equals a calm and relaxed body

Hospitals do not advise administering oxygen during labour unless there is a special circumstance, mainly because there isn't enough evidence to suggest that it is beneficial due to a lack of research in this area. In fact, a lack of oxygen within the pregnant body can cause distress in a baby, which can affect their heart rate and can cause a baby's heart rate to change which can indicate distress, a special circumstance that may therefore need intervention.

You and your baby also need a good supply of oxygen during pregnancy, as it helps with growth and development, so a lack of it can be potentially harmful. It is therefore important for you to avoid any behaviour that could reduce the amount of oxygen that you and your baby receive; for example, smoking and poor breathing habits.

No matter how well designed your body is to give birth, without oxygen you cannot expect it to do what you want it to do. It's a bit like attempting to drive a car without any fuel, it won't work!

Always remember: When you breathe the hypnobirthing way you can be sure that your uterus muscle is receiving a good supply of oxygen ensuring that your surges are as effective as they can be during your labour.

Chapter 12:

Design

Trust your body, it knows what to do!

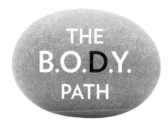

D – Design

Without the knowledge that is required to understand how your body works you will be unable to connect and take control of the powerful feelings associated with labour. What I am talking about is understanding the DESIGN of your incredible body.

In my hypnobirthing classes I often use props to demonstrate how the uterus muscle works, because I believe fully understanding the workings of this amazing muscle is the key to understanding childbirth.

I first fell in love with the physiology of the human body during my biology classes at school and it's one of the reasons why I decided to become a nurse. I love teaching how a woman's body is designed to birth as it explains the science behind it all. It is often the 'aha moment' part of the teaching that really resonates with many. Please don't just accept that your uterus muscle will know how to get your baby out. Understand how it is so cleverly designed and what it needs to do to get your baby out on the day. That way you will be more able to connect with the powerful feelings, embrace the feelings and even look forward to the feelings of labour.

Your uterus is known as your 'birthing muscle' and it's made up of two types of muscle fibres that need to work together in order for your cervix (the lowest part of the uterus) to become thinner and dilate, making way for your baby to then come down the birth path. It is important that you understand how your muscles will work for you on the day and your hypnobirthing techniques will enable you to fully embrace this vital part of the birth process.

When your uterus is relaxed it will be able to then do what it is perfectly designed to do, so that when it is time for your baby's head to apply pressure on your cervix, it will enable it to soften and open until it becomes fully dilated, allowing your baby to then move down the birth path. Your hypnobirthing teacher will show you how to achieve this easily and effortlessly when they help you to become an expert in relaxation.

Your pelvis

As well as knowing the ins and outs of this birthing muscle it is important to understand how incredibly well designed your pelvis is too. The female pelvis is like a bony cradle that rocks and protects your baby and is perfectly designed for giving birth. It is designed in such a way to carry the weight of both you and your baby, as well as helping to protect your internal organs. Another function of your amazing pelvis is to provide attachment for your abdominal muscles as well as the muscles of your pelvic floor. You might want to think about doing some pelvic floor exercises now too. More about that soon.

During labour, the ligaments of the pelvis will soften and stretch allowing the pelvis to widen and enable your baby to come down the birth path. Your pelvis is so very clever! You also have special hormones that are released which will cause the ligaments of your pelvis to soften, stretch and become flexible so that your baby's head can pass through during birth. The soft tissues of the pelvis will also help your baby to turn into the position that is right for them when the time is right. It is normal to feel some pelvic discomfort whilst pregnant due to the loosening of the joints, but if this discomfort becomes severe please consult with your caregiver for specific advice in this area.

When you know what to do to help move your coccyx (tailbone) out of the way during labour, you will be able to make more room for your baby to get into a better position and come down the birth path. Imagine trying to slide down a slide with a curled up end. It's likely that you will get stuck, making it difficult to go any further. Why some women are still encouraged to birth on their backs with their coccyx bone preventing their baby from moving down, I will never know!

Get up, get moving. It's all about your birthing positions which, of course, your hypnobirthing teacher will cover in class. I like to think of your pelvis as a protective, comfortable and well-feathered little nest perfectly designed for you and your baby.

We have spoken about the importance of understanding your physiology but you also need to understand the physiology of your baby; after all Mother Nature is clever and so is your baby.

Have you ever wondered how on earth a baby's head can have the ability to come out of a donut or bagel-shaped opening? I hope I haven't triggered a craving now, but have you? Well, your body is clever and so is your baby. When your baby comes down the birth path their head will reduce in circumference, meaning your baby's head will mould into a cone-like shape and become thinner making it easier for you to birth your baby. What a clever baby you have growing inside you!

A baby born by Caesarean section tends to have a more perfectly rounded head due to their alternate exit. A baby born this way may also breathe faster and shallower than a baby that has come down the birth path because of the surges in the womb as well as the compression of your baby's chest when coming down the birth path. Some babies can have cone-shaped heads for a few days or even longer because of squeezing down the birth path but most will return to normal in no time at all.

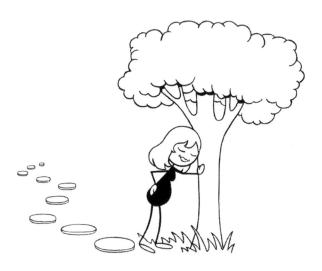

The above image shows the position you will want to adopt in labour because of the way your pelvis is designed. Your teacher will explain the many different labour positions to try in order to open your pelvis and allow gravity to assist the descent of your baby down the birth path.

The pelvic tilt

This position is useful throughout labour. The pelvic tilt position helps to not only ease any discomfort in your lower back, but also helps your baby to get into a good position for birthing. As you can see in the image above, this upright and forward position moves your coccyx bone out of the way, making more space for your baby to come down the birth path. Women who choose to have an epidural during labour are less likely to be able to adopt this position whilst birthing.

What will your baby feel?

Before your baby comes down the birth path the goal will be to provide them with plenty of oxytocin along the way. This will help them feel safe, content, calm and loved during this time.

I have always wondered what a baby feels when they come down the birth path and the only thing I can imagine it to be like is when you are getting in or out of your car when someone has parked too close to your door. You know that feeling when you need to suck it all in in order to get back into your car again? I wouldn't call this painful but maybe slightly uncomfortable. As I said, this is just my opinion and something I have always wondered.

What will your baby hear when they are coming down the birth path?

We know babies can hear because they have been communicating with you all along and can already recognise the sound of your voice. Your baby may be comforted by your voice in labour too, as well as the calming voice you will be listening to on your hypnobirthing tracks.

What will your baby see when they are coming down the birth path?

Obviously they have been in the dark up to this point and it's only when they are born that they will first experience blurry vision. If you were to hold your baby about 10–20 inches away from your face it can help them focus more easily on you. (This is also known as the birth imprint.) I have much more to share with you about the importance of this moment when it's time for you to explore the final path known as the B.A.B.Y. Path.

As your labour progresses, your baby will do all that they can to help in the process too. I clearly remember the moment when I could feel Alana nudging her way down; I was totally connected to her with a real sense of the two of us working together as one. Oh how I would love to relive that moment again if I could!

The Moment Of Birth

'Before my baby girl embarked on her journey down the birth path she was filled with excitement, knowing that she will finally be able to put faces to all those muffled voices that have gently spoken to her and comforted her along the way.

When the time was right she looked behind one last time at the warm and soothing cove that had bathed and allowed her to thrive into the being that she has become. She thanks her first home that she has now outgrown and she smiles reassuringly, knowing that a new home is waiting for her. Outside is a place she has dreamt of many times although the time has never felt right to explore those feelings until this very moment.

She is ready and eager to present herself to the world outside having travelled a long way in isolation, the bumps, the twists, the turns, the wonder of not knowing what anything is or what anything means, a serene place to simply explore, wonder and just be.

In front of her, she sees a path unfolding, so new and intriguing, knowing that to enter means no return; her home no longer, gone forever, but that's ok as it just feels right to now embark on this new and exciting journey.

The direction of the path is so clearly laid out in front of her, she experiences a gentle nudge of encouragement as she feels an ever so slight current developing within the ethereal waters that surround her.

She remains intrigued by the environmental changes around her and the innate force of nature that causes her to feel new and arousing emotions like she has never felt before. With intrinsic certainty, she is finally ready to make her way down the birth path as she hears my voice from within one last time. A vibrational humming sensation nudges her down giving her the confidence to allow herself to continue to follow the birth path with grace and ease.

She feels snug, arms and legs unable to move like they used to, the feeling of a soft but flexible wall surrounds her as she gently nudges down further.

She feels a fresh wave of air brush across the top of her head which startles her at first causing her heart to again change its beat. The path has slowed down a little and she rests to gather her thoughts before going any further. Her heart is beating faster now as the excitement of almost completing her journey nears.

"I can do this' she says, "I have come so far, I am excited to meet these voices, I am ready to be born", and with one last powerful surge her head slowly emerges. My baby, a girl! I finally have my girl. Alana Ruby will be her name.'

Tamara x

Your posture is important!

In today's society we tend to be much more sedentary; we have soft comfy sofas, bucket seats in cars and we are generally a lot less active. Research has shown that we have a lot more malpositioned babies because of this and therefore we know that the position of your baby is directly influenced by your posture. You can keep good posture by doing the following things:

• Sit up straight instead of slouching into the sofa.

• Use a birthing ball when resting.

• Getting on your hands and knees (a hammock-like position).

• Straddling a chair when sitting.

• Sit in positions where your knees are lower than your hips, and knees are pointing downward.

• Lean forward throughout the day and do some cat stretches (arched back).

'Something that really helped me remember good posture is whenever I sat down I would imagine a piece of string attached to the top of my head and in order to keep

the string hanging straight down I would focus on it reaching my chin, then the middle of my chest and then my belly button.'

Tamara x

Pelvic floor exercises

Being pregnant can place stress on your pelvic floor muscles. They are known as a 'sling' of muscles, a bit like a small muscle hammock that runs between the pubic bone in the front and the tailbone at the back. Your pelvic floor muscles support your womb (uterus), bladder, and bowel. Your pelvic floor can become weak and stretched from as early as 12 weeks into your pregnancy. It is also possible that those experiencing constipation, which is common in pregnant women, can put even more strain on their pelvic floor. The most difficult thing can be remembering to do your pelvic floor exercises (also known as kegels) so you may want to make them part of your daily routine.

A good way to remember is to set an anchor (a reminder) for yourself, i.e. Every time you brush your teeth you can pull up with your pelvic floor, or every time you pull up at a red light in a car you can pull up with your pelvic floor. What really helped me remember was to stick a post-it note on the dashboard of my car that read 'PFE'. Pelvic floor exercises, if done properly, can help to protect you from incontinence while you're pregnant as well as after your baby is born. Your hypnobirthing teacher will teach you in class how these exercises are done properly.

Always remember: Fully understanding how your body works and why you are designed the way you are will help you connect with the powerful feelings associated with birth. Hypnobirthing will help you connect with your incredible body so that the feelings of birthing are better understood and feel more natural to you.

Chapter 13:

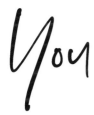

Your positive birth is on the other side of fear!

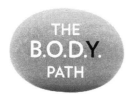

Y – You

It's now time to explore the last step in the B.O.D.Y. Path. If you don't embrace this step there really is no point going any further. If you don't dig deep and explore this area you will be unable to find the freedom YOU need to open your mind and find the answers to why you think and feel the way you do; and the same applies to your birth partner too.

When you do understand this fundamental area in greater detail you will be more able to accept the challenges or obstacles that can come your way throughout pregnancy. Hypnobirthing will help you feel less stressed and less worried, knowing that you have done all you can to face your fears head on.

I am sure by now you have a better understanding of where your thoughts about childbirth have come from and that I have pressed enough buttons in your thought process to make that happen. Giving yourself permission to just sit and think for a while so that YOU could explore your feelings has been much of my focus. I trust that YOU have discovered some really useful information about yourself so far.

I shared with you my personal experience of where my beliefs came from earlier and maybe this is an area that you might want to spend some time exploring for yourself. You might not even have the answers right now and that's fine. When you attend a hypnobirthing course it will help you find the answers and show you how you can manage or even overcome your worries or fears.

You and your baby deserve to experience a pregnancy that is calm and relaxed, without the constant niggling of negative thoughts about what could happen on the day. I have always wondered why some people worry more than others or is it simply down to the way you are wired? I can understand the need to worry if something has happened that is worth worrying about. If nothing has happened however, and it's just your creative thoughts getting in the way, then you will need some tools to manage them.

Hypnobirthing teaches you very simple yet very effective techniques that will help take your mind off anything that may be causing you to feel worried or stressed. These techniques are not just for birth and can therefore be applied to other areas of your life too which is great for you and your birth partner, not to mention great value on the investment that you make when you join a hypnobirthing course.

Hypnobirthing will teach YOU tools for life

Over the many years that I have taught hypnobirthing I have discovered that these tools for life can be used in so many different ways. Here is a list of experiences that couples have shared with me about their continued use of their hypnobirthing techniques after the birth of their baby:

- *'I used the breathing and imagining my relaxing place in nature whilst visiting the dentist.'*

- *'I still use the music to soothe my baby and I watch him settle instantly.'*

- *'I did the breathing techniques just before the job interview and it kept me calm.'*

- *'I really don't like trains so when I feel anxiety coming on I just use the breathing I learnt.'*

- *'I never road rage anymore, I just take a deep breath and slow my breathing down.'*

- *'I still use the same smell when having a bath because I love to reminisce.'*

- *'I close my eyes and imagine the ocean when having blood tests.'*

- *'I needed a smear test so I just focused on my breathing to relax.'*

- *'I still love listening to the music, I feel relaxed whenever I put it on.'*

If you're anything like me and dislike blood tests and dentists then you can use the techniques to help with any anxiety you might experience in your daily life. Let's look at anxiety and how it can affect you in labour. If you go through pregnancy with persistent worry and fear about what 'might happen' in labour and birth it can cause your body to experience what's known as the flight, fight, freeze, faint response.

YOU might flight, fight, freeze or faint

It's actually a survival mechanism that all human beings have to keep us alive and keep us safe from dangerous situations. You will need to learn how to avoid your body going into this detrimental state during labour.

The reason for this is because the flight, fight, freeze, faint response within your body is one of the main causes of complications in labour and birth as it can slow down labour and cause distress in both you and your baby. You need to do everything you can to prevent your fears from getting in the way and avoid this involuntary response happening to you during your labour and birth.

I have suffered from anxiety in the past and I wouldn't wish it on anyone. It feels like your heart is about to jump out of your chest with a real sense of losing control. It's a horrible feeling and I learnt how to deal with this through breathing. Even now if I start to feel nervous or apprehensive in a situation I will focus on my breathing techniques and the feeling will go away. As I said, these techniques will become tools for life for you.

I said it before and I'll say it again

Some people are influenced by the information around them more so than others; some question it and some simply accept it, not knowing that they are actually being influenced at a subconscious level. This is the part of your mind where your beliefs are stored and I am happy to say that yes, your beliefs can be changed, but only if YOU want to change them. You have everything within you to change your beliefs around childbirth, and the knowledge contained within this book, in conjunction with your hypnobirthing teacher to guide you along the way, will ensure you make those necessary changes.

FEAR – A poem by Khalil Gibran

It is said that before entering the sea
a river trembles with fear.

She looks back at the path she has travelled,
from the peaks of the mountains,
the long winding road crossing forests and villages.

And in front of her,
she sees an ocean so vast,
that to enter
there seems nothing more than to disappear forever.

But there is no other way.
The river cannot go back.

Nobody can go back.
To go back is impossible in existence.

The river needs to take the risk
of entering the ocean
because only then will fear disappear,
because that's where the river will know
it's not about disappearing into the ocean,
but of becoming the ocean.

The physiology of birth and the impact of fear

So let's get straight to it and find out why so many women share such horror stories of birth and why it doesn't have to be that way. A question first! Assuming that there is no injury or excessive physical exertion, why do you think clever old Mother Nature is happy for all muscles of the body to function without discomfort, except the muscles of the uterus?

The good news is that the muscles of the uterus do work in the same way as all of our other muscles and let's look at how. The uterus is a muscular bag made up of involuntary muscles. Unlike the muscles that control the movement of your limbs, you cannot choose when these muscles work and therefore you can't strengthen them beforehand through exercise. Instead, the presence of the hormone oxytocin in sufficient quantities will ensure that these involuntary muscles surge in a regular pattern as required during labour. The involuntary muscles of the uterus are divided into two types just as I mentioned earlier when looking at the design of your amazing body.

The outer longitudinal (vertical) muscles known as the active segment and the inner circular (relaxed) muscles found mainly at the lower part of the uterus and known as the passive segment. During dilation, the vertical muscles draw up the relaxed circular muscles whilst also pushing the baby's head against the cervix. The repeated pressure of the baby's head on the cervix causes the cervix to thin out and then retract around the baby's head. You are considered to be fully dilated at 10cm, as this is the average size of a baby's head, and the baby is then ready to make their way down the birth path.

You will learn all about the birthing phase later on when you visit the B.A.B.Y. Path. As mentioned previously, the inner circular muscles are meant to be relaxed and passive during a surge in order for the vertical muscles to work effectively, however this is not always the case.

Your hypnobirthing teacher will demonstrate in class exactly how your uterus will work for you using specific exercises, images and creative props to help with your learning.

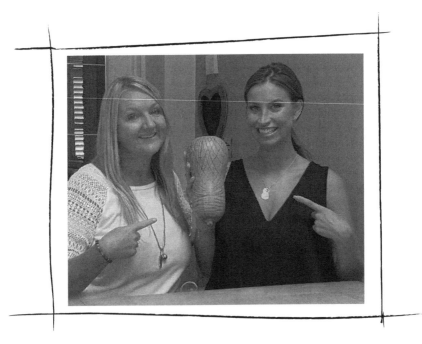

Television presenter and celebrity Ferne McCann at 29 weeks pregnant learned all about her amazing body using my butternut squash. Ferne of course said: 'The only way is hypnobirthing!'

Cervix is closed, cervix is opening

The impact of fear on the labouring woman is intense. When a woman goes into labour with any fear, is stressed or anxious, or circumstances arise during her labour that create these emotional responses, stressor hormones called catecholamines are triggered. The one that is most important to us is adrenaline. The presence of adrenaline sets off what we know as the 'fight, flight, faint or freeze' response.

This subconscious, automatic, inborn response that occurs when we are faced with danger, gives us the strength to stand and fight, run away, faint or (left with no other choice) freeze i.e. feign death and hope that the danger passes us by. When this occurs, the blood vessels contract in most of the body, redirecting the blood toward the heart, lungs and major muscle groups to help fuel the reaction.

This in turn causes oxygen to move away from the uterus and indeed the baby. Non-essential body systems are put on hold and this includes the uterus muscle. With adrenaline present and causing a lack of oxygen in the uterus, the inner circular muscles are now no longer relaxed, but the vertical muscles keep pulling them up (you can imagine why this would cause pain).

In turn, the vertical muscles become overworked (much like when we do too many reps at the gym) so they too are beginning to cause pain. Adrenaline also inhibits the production of endorphins, our body's natural pain relief.

The impact of fear on the baby

Lack of oxygen in the uterus means a lack of oxygen for the baby and this, combined with the continual pressure of the baby's head against a now taut cervix, can lead the baby to become distressed. The adrenaline (the 'OMG I'm gonna die!' hormone) reduces oxytocin levels causing surges to slow down or even stop altogether. With dilation not happening as quickly as the medical team might like, resulting in a distressed baby, you see the potential for intervention taking place and natural labour being less likely.

Why does this happen?

Why on earth, if the body is so clever, would it do that, you might be thinking? Quite simply, it comes down to survival. This is best explained through the eyes of an animal. Suddenly a predator comes on the scene and the last thing the mummy animal wants to do is provide it with an easy target for lunch. The fear response within her causes the constriction to occur which enables her to move to a place of safety. Once she is completely sure that she is safe again, her body returns to normal and she continues to birth her baby comfortably. Isn't nature clever?

If your cat has ever had kittens, you would have noticed that the place they choose to birth in will be a warm, dark, quiet environment where they can feel safe. Now, if mummy cat perceives a dangerous situation her labour will stop until she feels safe again and will then continue to birth her kittens. You will need to feel safe and secure in your birthing environment too and this is where your hypnobirthing techniques come in.

There are a number of important factors to consider in order to help prevent adrenaline being present during your baby's birth:

- Address any fears you may have in terms of both your baby's birth and becoming a parent prior to having your baby.

- Ensure you feel 'safe' and spend time researching your birthing options.

I have always found it interesting that the letters FTP (fear, tension, pain) are also what medical professionals use to describe some women in labour who are not progressing. They will often use the term FTP (failure to progress). Breathing the hypnobirthing way will help you relax and reduce the intensity of the feeling. Just a reminder here again that hypnobirthing will not guarantee you a pain-free birth but it will promote a more comfortable state of mind and body.

Thank you fear, but I no longer need YOU in my life

'Something to firstly ask yourself is, "Where's this fear coming from?" Are they patterns you learned as a young child? You may have these patterns that you developed, these mechanisms you developed because at the time you were searching for love or safety and you created these coping mechanisms. Maybe one of those mechanisms was "fear"'.

Are you always looking for those threats, the threats that you are going to have a horrible birth experience? And maybe if you can find those patterns you can look at that pattern, this fear of a horrible birth or this fear of whatever, and ask, 'How does that serve me? How has it served me in the past? How has it helped me in the past?' Honour that fear, that feeling, and ask, 'How is it going to help me if I leave the fear behind?'

Feeling this way may have served you in the past, but it's not going to serve you going forward. Hypnobirthing will help you to let it go. Focus on change and where you are going when you leave that feeling behind you.'

Tamara x

How do YOU relax?

I am sure that you will have your own ideas about what relaxation means to you. But I tend to find that when I ask parents this question, the general response is 'mind empty, body still', or something similar. For some this is perfectly fine, for others it creates the complete opposite of what you are aiming to achieve, and that is tension or anxiety. They will say things such as 'I don't relax well' or, 'My mind never switches off' or, 'I can never sit still'.

Well, the good news is that you don't need to have an empty mind or a completely still body in order to move into a deep state of relaxation. In fact, if you spent your time 'trying' to be still then you would be creating tension in the body, and if you worry about creating an empty mind you are less likely to let go of conscious thought. So, both are completely counterproductive.

Certainly, during labour, the last thing I would want is for a mum to feel that she must be still the whole time, as it is important for a labouring woman to follow her instincts and what her body needs.

Very often, particularly in the earlier stages of labour, women are drawn to being more upright and active. You may want to rock on a birthing ball or lean forward against a wall or tree if out on a walk. Often during a hypnosis session, someone will get so lost in their inner thoughts that their body will become completely still; but as we don't stay still even when we are asleep, there really is no reason why an adjustment would affect the experience.

In fact no adjustment would affect the experience, if it is desired. What we are looking for is emotional relaxation. Of course, if the mind is calm the body can only follow, but we can be lost in our thoughts whilst taking a lovely walk, feeling completely relaxed and happy. Eyes open, body active but in a complete state of trance, not caring to notice too much of what is going on around us. For me personally, playing a sport has always been what relaxes me. The more physical the sport the more I am able to switch off to everything around me. This is why I chose to play Roller Derby for many years. My team would even prepare for a big game by listening to my hypnosis tracks to build confidence and calm any pre-game nerves. This is another great example of how these tools can be used in other aspects of your life. You really won't know whether you will want to remain still or be more active in labour when the time comes because birthing is so instinctive.

What position will help YOU relax best?

The simple answer to this is to follow what your body is telling you. Seek to be as comfortable as you can be on whatever surface you are resting on. This is because if for any reason you are not completely comfortable, due to either physical causes or because the surface upon which you are resting isn't the best it can be, there will be conflict in your mind. You can always be as comfortable as you can be, and by setting this intention you will enable your subconscious mind to let go more easily. I have always found that practising relaxation in lots of different positions and in different rooms of the house, even the garden, is a great way to practise because you just don't know where or what your body will want to do until that time comes.

Did YOU know that distractions can be useful?

You won't be able to completely control what is happening around you, or even within you, when you are practising your hypnobirthing skills, so it is useful to understand how to let go of distractions. The subconscious mind naturally has to filter out information, focusing only on what it believes is important at any given moment. Without this we would not be able to cope. Because it does this, we know that we too can consciously decide what is important and what is not. Should you have any sensations in the body during trance, an itch, a desire to move your hair or adjust your body, respond to that and make adjustments as appropriate. To 'try' and ignore these urges can prevent relaxation and possibly cause further distraction.

As we've mentioned before, you will not want to be still all the time whilst in labour, so it is useful to acknowledge that movement will not distract you from the deep state of relaxation you are in. Should any unwanted sounds occur simply say to yourself, 'the sounds around me help me to become more internally focused.' Just like you don't hear the hum of others talking in a busy street when you are chatting with your friends, so you can send any unwanted sounds into the background whilst enjoying and using your hypnobirthing tools and techniques.

When you relax, your endorphins are stimulated, which is such a lovely feeling for your baby and may cause you to think that they will become more relaxed too, i.e. less active. It may surprise you then to find that often they become more active which is due to your muscles softening and therefore creating more room for them to stretch, move about and kick out. Enjoy your baby's movements, knowing that they are enjoying themselves, and let it simply become part of your pregnancy experience.

As we walked through the doors of the delivery suite the fire alarms went off. The midwife hurried us to a room and immediately apologised for the loud noise. Sam instinctively got onto her hands and knees and closed her eyes. The fire alarm lasted around 2 minutes but what we didn't expect was for it to go off on the hour, every hour after that. As Sam's doula there wasn't anything I could do about it and I remember just hoping that it didn't effect her too much. It was so loud and every time the bell rang I would feel my heart jump out of my chest. On reflection, Sam said that she wasn't really that bothered by the constant alarms throughout and just focused on her breathing. She mentioned that whenever she heard the alarm she would simply say to herself, "the sound of the alarm takes me further into relaxation." A well-trained hypnobirthing mummy indeed and a great example of how distractions can be perceived as useful triggers to deepen relaxation even more'.

Tamara x

What will a 'uterine surge' feel like to YOU?

Some women want to know in advance what a surge is going to feel like but really that is like asking 'how long is a piece of string?'. As I've already discussed, every person experiences sensations differently and uniquely, so even when a person describes what something is like for them, it doesn't mean it will be like that for you.

The most important feeling you can focus on during your practice is what being comfortable feels like to you. I can be clearer about where women experience a surge and you may find it surprising to learn that this is not necessarily around the tummy. Some women in labour feel the sensations in their abdomen and others in their lower back or even their thighs. That said, I appreciate I may still not have appeased some of your curiosity and so I've shared some of the unique interpretations that I have received in the past.

Every woman is different!

'My surges felt like powerful tightening sensations, quite high up in my abdomen.'

'My surge felt like a pulling sensation in my lower abdomen.'

'I experienced a burrowing-down sensation.'

'My surges felt like waves of pressure in my tummy.'

'My bump went rock hard every time I experienced a surge.'

'I felt every surge in my thighs only, this was most unexpected.'

'The only place I felt the surge was in my lower back and it was extremely intense.'

'I just felt pressure, no pain, just pressure.'

Self-hypnosis (YOU will achieve this relaxed state all by yourself)

All formal hypnosis is in fact self-hypnosis whether you are in a face-to-face class with your hypnobirthing teacher or listening to a hypnosis track using your own inner thoughts. This is because you are ALWAYS in control. Your hypnobirthing teacher will guide you towards finding a relaxing place in nature that is just right for you. This is a safe place that you can visit in your mind anytime you want to. It can be a made-up place, or an actual location of somewhere you've enjoyed or would like to go to. Or you may wish to visit a holiday destination, relaxing by the ocean or somewhere else in nature. Making your way to a relaxing place provides direction and somewhere that can occupy your mind, leaving your body and baby to do what they need to do, unhindered by any conscious interference.

Did YOU know you can do this with your eyes open too?

Because you enter the trance state naturally and much of the time you are doing this you will have your eyes open (daydreaming, engrossed in a good movie, new lovers entranced by each other, etc.), you can also maintain a state of hypnosis without having to lie still with your eyes closed. In fact, for birthing this is a very important thing to be aware of because you will find that particularly during the early stages you will most probably have the urge to be quite active.

Now that you have a better understanding of hypnosis, it is time to start practising with your eyes open and moving about, as well as whilst you are resting back with them closed. The more you practise with your eyes open, the easier that trance-like state will become. The goal is to be able to do this any time, any place, anywhere.

Time flies when you're having fun!

You naturally distort time; waiting in a queue at the checkout may only take five minutes but it can seem like ages. That same five minutes when at a party having fun will zoom by in a flash. Of course, if you are bored at the party it will drag and if you are chatting with your friend in the queue you will be paying before you know it. This is particularly useful during labour. A woman who is focusing on nothing but dreading each surge will cause them to feel like they are coming quicker. If whilst experiencing each surge you give them 100% of your attention, you will naturally drag the time out. When you become more deeply relaxed or even go so far as to say you're enjoying yourself with the help from your hypnobirthing techniques, you will be less aware of how time is passing. My hypnobirth was six hours in total but the entire experience felt like two hours because I was enjoying myself so much, and this is something that hypnobirthing parents report back to me often.

Hypnobirthing will show YOU how to use 'anchors' to enhance relaxation

An anchor is a technique where you condition a sensory stimulus to a positive feeling or state of mind. You naturally anchor emotions through your senses whether that be smell, sound etc. Anchors occur naturally or can be set up like you will learn in class. When you establish an anchor in trance, it translates later in regular awareness to trigger associated suggestions, reactions and in this case relaxation.

• The following are some examples of what I mean by anchoring;

• Think about your favourite song and how it makes you feel?

- Does your partner wear a particular perfume/aftershave? If you smell it, what feelings does it bring up for you? As you pass through an area in which you had a great childhood experience, how does it make you feel? This can also happen with negative feelings, depending on what the anchor is.

- If you have been ill after eating a particular food, what sensations do you get in your body when you think about this food?

Knowing that you do this naturally is very useful for you, because it means you can create useful anchors that you can trigger anytime you need them. When you are birthing you will want to create anchors to deepen your relaxation using mainly smell, sound and your birth partner's voice and touch.

Using smells or scents to enhance relaxation is powerful because we naturally anchor smells; if you are particularly fond of a certain fragrance then you can use this as an additional trigger for relaxation. Use it whenever you practise your relaxation techniques and you will create a strong associational link between the smell and a deep state of relaxation.

Tip: If you are choosing an essential oil firstly check that it is safe to use by asking a trained aromatherapist. Get yourself a cup of hot water and add a few drops in it. This is a great alternative to oil burners which of course you cannot take into a hospital (You cannot light a flame in a hospital due to the oxygen on the walls).

Tamara x

> Always remember: You will continue to use all that you will learn in your everyday life. Hypnobirthing will remove your fears and empower you with effective techniques to remain calm and relaxed during the birth of your baby. Hypnobirthing will give you the control back.

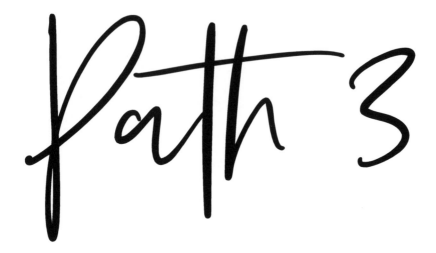

The B.R.E.A.T.H. Path

The B.R.E.A.T.H. Path

The breath is the link between the mind and the body

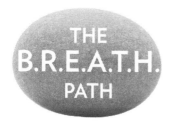

Knowing how to **BREATHE** the hypnobirthing way is what will get you through one of the most important days of your life. The hypnobirthing **RELAXATION** techniques will keep you calm, relaxed and in control in a nurtured **ENVIRONMENT** that makes you feel safe and secure. Knowing when and how to **APPLY** your hypnobirthing techniques is vital alongside making time to **TRAIN** and to practise. **HORMONES** play a major part in the birth process so you will need to know about how they work too.

Chapter 14:

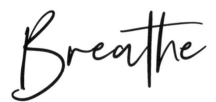

How you breathe will determine how you feel and how you birth

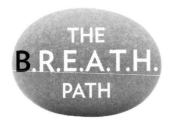

B – Breathe

The first step in the B.R.E.A.T.H. Path is all about your breathing. Have you ever noticed what happens to your breath when you become anxious or scared? It becomes faster and shallower doesn't it? This is the trigger for your body to go into the freeze, flight, fight, faint response I mentioned earlier making it vital that you learn how to manage this state.

Understanding and knowing how to BREATHE will be your antidote to this powerful physical response that can occur during labour. If you don't learn how to breathe properly in labour you will more easily feel out of control in labour, meaning the hormones associated with the freeze, flight, fight, faint response will increase causing your heart rate and breathing rate to become more rapid.

The hormone within your body that is responsible for this is known as adrenaline. Think back to a time in your life where something happened suddenly to cause you to feel frightened or shocked. The first physical response you may have noticed in your body was that your heart was beating a lot faster than it was a few seconds before the event; it's the adrenaline that causes your body to respond like this.

The quickest fix for being scared is knowing how to breathe properly. Therefore it is an absolute MUST that you master your hypnobirthing breathing techniques as soon as you can. As a doula I find myself often reminding mums how to breathe if they start to lose focus and it's amazing to witness with only a few words of encouragement how she is able to bring herself back into a calm state and regulate her breathing pattern again, giving her control back over her birth. Your hypnobirthing teacher will direct your partner in a similar way so that they can support you if you happen to go off track.

'Learning how to breathe was one of the most useful techniques I learnt during my pregnancy. I still remember that first surge and describing it just like an incredible force of nature. It's amazing how, when labour starts, you just know what to do. There were a couple of surges where I forgot to breathe properly and I really felt the difference in intensity. As soon as I went back to the hypnobirthing breath I coped so much better. I definitely put my confidence down to my daily hypnobirthing practice and the support of my partner as she knew exactly what to say to keep me going. Every woman needs to know how to do this!' – Emma and Fiona, first-time parents, London

Here are the top 10 reasons why you need to master your breath in labour

1 Knowing how to breathe properly helps to detox and release toxins within your body.

2 Breathing boosts your energy, stamina levels and elevates your mood.

3 Giving attention to your breathing increases your oxygen supply and relaxes your mind and body.

4 When you focus on your breath it can bring insight and clarity to you.

5 If you are feeling emotional, breathing can relieve any uneasy feelings.

6 Breathing relieves pain by breathing into it.

7 When you inhale, your abdomen will expand giving your uterus muscle plenty of oxygen.

8 You can improve your posture whilst pregnant with specific breathing techniques.

9 Deep breathing removes carbon dioxide and increases blood quality.

10 Breathing a certain way can release any stress or tension within your body, helping you to relax.

When we are calm, breathing slows down and creates more peace within us by its slow rhythmical movement. Paying attention to our breath brings us totally into the present moment. We can only breathe in the 'now', therefore when a labouring woman focuses on her breathing, she is unable to fixate on anything else that is happening. Will the surges become too intense, if she can't cope? This can create more fear, shallow breathing and a constriction of the uterine muscles, making labour much more difficult to manage.

Understanding this, the breath becomes one of the easiest ways to help us to relax the mind and body together and in turn our ability to remain calm, relaxed and in control throughout labour and birth. Because breathing changes when you are scared, if you practise deep, slow rhythmic breathing at times when you are relaxed and calm, we are more able to use the breath to keep calm and in control should upsetting situations arise, or indeed to avoid them occurring.

In between your surges you will learn how you can use your breath simply and easily to calm your mind and relax your body. You will learn how to take control of your breath, ensuring that during labour you will feel confident in your ability to trust your instincts and adapt what you have learnt. Should you start to experience Braxton Hicks (practice labour) you can use them as a signal to practise your breathing techniques.

Always remember: Hypnobirthing breathing is the most powerful way to redirect your focus during your surges and at the same time ensure that your body remains relaxed. This is the key when it comes to your uterus doing what it needs to do whilst birthing. Knowing how to breathe in a particular way is the vital ingredient.

Chapter 15:

Relaxation

Choose to relax….it feels better!

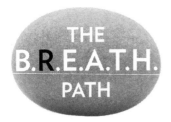

R – Relaxation

The next step in the B.R.E.A.T.H. Path happens to be the direct effect of mastering your breathing techniques. It is important to understand this step because without knowing how to achieve this, it will prevent your body and mind from doing what they need to do in labour. When you learn how to achieve this state you will notice that you will be able to remain calm, focused and in control during your pregnancy and labour. What I am talking about is understanding and learning the art of RELAXATION.

If you were to approach an out of control woman in labour and suggest that she calms down and relaxes she won't be able to unless she has previously taught herself how to do this. I know that if I am angry about something (which doesn't happen often because I am a relaxation expert, after all) and someone tells me to calm down, it makes me even angrier.

I have seen women in labour become extremely frustrated when either their partner or midwife tells them to calm down. How can you calm down if you don't know how to? This is where your hypnobirthing techniques come in. Just knowing that you must be relaxed on the day when you birth your baby is not enough! You need to practise relaxation so that you can go in and out of this state as and when you need. In my experience as a doula, mums who have been able to achieve a relaxed state in labour not only enjoy the experience more but their labours are shorter and easier.

I have also attended births where mums haven't been able to achieve a relaxed state and although they reported back that labour was challenging for them, they still described their labour and birth as a positive experience because of the knowledge they received when attending their hypnobirthing course. I would love to be able to promise you a relaxed labour and birth but unfortunately I can't. I can, however, tell you that by attending a hypnobirthing course and practising the techniques, you will be giving yourself the best chance of achieving the right birth on the day.

Your hypnobirthing teacher will teach you how to relax on your own, anywhere and at any time both physically and emotionally. When relaxed in labour you will be able to focus and concentrate better, become more present in the moment and have a better memory of your experience when you reflect on your special day afterwards. When you are relaxed and focused, you will have better clarity over the decisions that you will need to make on the day and they will be informed decisions, rather than feeling like you were forced down a route you really didn't want to take.

When you are relaxed you will be able to think more clearly and ask the appropriate questions regarding the direction that your labour and birth is going in… and so will your birth partner! If you do not learn how to relax you will experience more pain! Yes, I know that sounds harsh but it is a fact! Women who are stressed and frightened during labour do experience more pain and quite often longer labours too. I have already mentioned why this is; remember when you learnt about how fear can affect your body in labour? By learning how to relax your muscles you will reduce any physical tension and pain and have more control over your state of mind. When your muscles are relaxed it is more difficult to worry, and when your mind is relaxed you will be more able to think positive thoughts on the day too.

Learning the art of relaxation will give you more energy in all areas of your life. When your body feels better, your mind will be focused and you will function better. Your baby will love the feeling they get when you relax too because you are completely connected with your baby both physically and emotionally.

If you could see your baby's face when you are in a relaxed state I bet they would be smiling. You might even find that your baby becomes more active when you relax, so just enjoy the movements of your baby saying how much they too love the feeling of relaxation. There is no better reason than to master relaxation now for you and your baby! I have a beautiful relaxation technique set in a lovely relaxing environment that I share on my courses. All my mums and their babies love it! I'm sure your hypnobirthing teacher will have one too.

'As I lay there on my side in a deep state of relaxation, listening to my relaxation tracks, I remember a doctor coming into my room and in a loud voice asked what blood group I was in case I needed a blood transfusion. I remember thinking who is this woman and how dare she come into my room and disturb me like this. I opened my eyes, stared at her and said 'I'm B positive'. I then closed my eyes and went back to my relaxing place in my mind. I only knew this because I had needed a blood transfusion after my son's birth but also what a perfect response to her question. What I found out later is that my mum, who was there with me on the day, pretty much pushed that doctor out the door for rudely interrupting me like this. The main thing to take away from this story (apart from not to mess with my mum) is how hypnobirthing can give you the ability to quickly and easily get yourself back into the zone again if something happens suddenly that requires your attention.'

Tamara x

Always remember: Hypnobirthing will turn you into an expert in relaxation. Learning how to relax now and in the future will enable you to make better decisions on your birthing day and as a parent too. Hypnobirthing parents often report that what they learnt in class was responsible for creating a calm and relaxed baby.

Chapter 16:

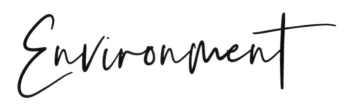

Environment

Surround yourself with things that make you happy!

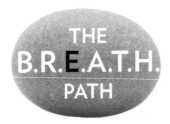

THE B.R.E.A.T.H. PATH

E – Environment

It's now time to talk about where and how you are planning to birth your baby. As far as I am concerned, couples who spend time ensuring that this is as perfect as it can be, birth far more easily. The 'E' in the B.R.E.A.T.H. Path represents the very important ENVIRONMENT that your baby will be born in.

Feeling safe as a birthing woman is vital as this will affect the way you feel throughout, particularly when it comes to remaining confident and feeling supported so that you can relax and focus on implementing your hypnobirthing techniques.

Whether you feel safe during your birth experience will depend on the level of stress experienced. Hospitals are changing, with more and more refurbishments including pools, mood lighting and nature murals on the walls, but many still remain relatively clinical environments. This birthing environment needs to minimise stress and facilitate the physiology of labour and birth, thereby contributing to a safe and satisfying birth experience for all.

The hospital birth environment is a foreign place and can provoke fear and anxiety. This can interrupt the delicate hormonal influences that drive labour and birth, making intervention more likely. It is wonderful to see that more and more birth spaces are being designed to feel safe and calming. Midwives and doulas are witnessing reduced intervention rates and more positive birth experiences when the birthing environment is seriously considered.

When identifying what is important in the birthing environment it is vital to look at the design of the room and what is included. Is there privacy, a bed, a pool, dim lighting, private shower/bath/toilet, quietness, windows, temperature controls, other furniture, space to move around, positive images, easy access, calming smells and most importantly supportive people?

The overall focus is on the creation of a space in which women are most likely to feel safe and relaxed during labour and birth. Such an environment is characterised by privacy and homeliness, and provides the woman with a sense of personal control. Specifically:

- Doors and windows should be positioned and covered or screened so as to protect the privacy of the birthing woman.

- Furniture should encourage and support women to adopt a more upright position for labour and birth.

- A bath, suitable for water immersion, should be available in all birth rooms.

I often describe the birth partners in my class as silverback gorillas. I don't teach partners to bang on their chests or stamp their feet unless they really have to, of course. But if you look at the way a silverback protects his family in the wild, you'll see that he will do everything in his power to ensure that his family is safe. They are the protectors of the birthing environment with no one allowed to come near their mate.

Why not take on this archetype? I say to my class, 'But do make sure you allow your midwife to take blood pressure and listen to baby's heart rate.' It's a great analogy and quite often there is a dad sitting in class with his arms folded for me to point out the likeness of a gorilla to help make my point here. We do enjoy a giggle!

Why not birth in the same environment in which you conceived your baby?

Maybe there was slow, soft music in the background; candles were glowing, creating a peaceful dim light all around you with a lovely sensual scent in the air. If you are smiling now then you can see how an environment like this would be perfect for you to birth your baby in. We need to feel comfortable, safe and secure in the environment in which we birth, in order to birth more easily. Here is a list of things to think about that may affect the way you feel in the environment that you are birthing in:

- Who is in the room with you? You must feel comfortable with everyone in the room.

- Do you have a preferred smell that you may have been using whilst listening to your relaxations?

- Have a playlist of relaxing music and your hypnobirthing tracks.

- How would you like the lighting to be? If the lights can't be dimmed, some women like to cover their eyes with their hands or wear an eye mask whilst relaxing.

- Birthing ball, birthing stool, gym mats.

- Pool (for a water birth).

- En suite facilities.

As I've explained, if an animal birthing their young is faced with a situation where a predator is nearing, they will stop birthing until they find a safe place to continue. Human beings are the same in this respect, and if our environment is causing anxiety we can experience a labour that may slow down, stall or weaken.

During labour, your birthing partner will do what they can to ensure that there is nothing within your environment that could cause you emotional upset. However, when this is not possible, please remember that you are in charge of how you choose to react to something.

You are practising tools that will enable you to let go of your external environment whenever you need. If your external environment isn't as perfect as you'd like it to be and it cannot be changed, your birth partner can support you with utilising your hypnobirthing techniques instead. By focusing in this way you will still be able to remain calm, relaxed and in control, whatever is happening around you. One of the things I love about hypnobirthing is when you close your eyes and go within, regardless of the environment that you are in, your focus will be on diverting your mind to your happy place. I wonder whether you will have a little beach baby like I did?

Anything is possible when you surround yourself with supportive birth partners

The most important thing for a birth partner to understand is their role on the day. Mums, you will also want to let them know what your expectations are. I have broken these down into a number of categories.

Simple nurturing

Your birth partner will give you water and snacks whenever you need. If you have not moved for a while then they will check in with you to ensure that you are as comfortable as you can be. Suggesting a change in position can also be helpful. Other parts of their role include:

- Being your own personal DJ – making sure the right tracks are playing.

- Reminding you to go to the loo (a full bladder may affect the birth process).

- They will ensure that the environment is as perfect as it can be.

- Your partner will remain calm and make sure that you remain undisturbed as much as possible.

- They will support you with your relaxation through words and touch.

- Partners learn simple massage techniques to enhance your comfort.

- They will remind you of your techniques if you go off track.

Through words

In the same way that you will find your hypnobirthing techniques reassuring, if your partner speaks to you in a calm, relaxed, quiet way during labour, using soothing prompts at appropriate times, this can also help you to feel calm and relaxed. These can be as simple as 'you are doing great', 'I love you', I'm so proud of you', 'our baby is coming', 'it's so wonderful'. There are words (anchors) that your partner can use to enhance relaxation also, and you will learn this together in class.'

Supporting you with your relaxation techniques

Facial relaxation – if there is any tension in your face your partner can remind you to place the tip of your tongue behind your front upper teeth, or stroke your jaw and ask you to give a gentle smile or shush out a breath.

Positive signs for you and your partner to look out for during labour

- Any spotting of blood indicates that your body is directing its efforts downwards.

- Your body temperature may rise and/or drop alternately and one minute you might be kicking off your blanket and in another you might be requesting it back again. Experiencing cold feet is also common during labour, so pack warm socks.

- The need to open your bowels is a common feeling during labour.

- You may feel nausea or even feel the need to vomit; not nice I know but it can be a positive sign that your labour is progressing.

- Even the calmest of women sometimes get an urge to escape or declare that they cannot carry on. This sign is actually one of the most exciting as it often means that the moment of birth is just around the corner.

> Always remember: A woman needs to feel safe and secure in her birthing environment. Hypnobirthing parents know how to create the best possible environment to birth their baby in, whether that be in the comfort of your own home or in a hospital setting.

Chapter 17:

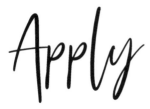

Knowing is not enough, you must learn how to apply this breath

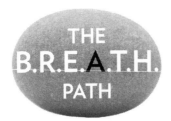

A – Apply

The next part of this path is all about APPLYING what you learn. Do you know what you want, and how to get it? Will you apply yourself and your knowledge? Will you see it through? Are you ready to do it? Or will you just contemplate it? There is no point doing a hypnobirthing course without full intentions of applying what you will learn on the day. Knowing about hypnobirthing is not enough; you need to attend a course so that you and your partner can work together so that you can apply the knowledge effectively and in a way that is just right for you.

The science behind the hypnobirthing breathing techniques

Is there any scientific basis for the proposed stress-relieving effects of a slow, deep, controlled breath? Let's begin with an exercise and then delve into the physiology behind your breathing. Find somewhere comfortable to sit and be mindful of your posture; bring your chest forward, allowing your shoulders to gently drop down. Relax your gaze and rest your hands comfortably in your lap. Now breathe into your abdomen, allowing your belly to fill up and expand on inhalation, pause momentarily and then slowly exhale, feeling your tummy slowly deflate as you do this.

Inhale through your nose for a slow count of four. Then exhale through your nose for a slow count of six.

Now close your eyes and repeat this process five times.

Rather than getting caught up in the numbers, however, it is best to just take slow, deep breaths, emphasising your change to the out breath.

Your body is constantly trying to maintain equilibrium. When you inhale, blood is drawn from your heart into your lungs. This creates a relative deficit of blood for the rest of your body. Your heart compensates by increasing the heart rate and pushing more blood and oxygen to your body.

How did this breath make you feel? Calm, happy, grounded, or maybe you have a better word to describe how you feel? Nevertheless, when your hypnobirthing teacher asks you to take a deep breath, smile, breathe deeply, and heed their wise advice because it really can make all the difference to the way you feel in the moment and of course when you are birthing your baby.

Applying relaxation around your mouth is important too

Throughout your practice you will be encouraged to relax your jaw. Any tension in your jaw can create tension in your pelvic area. Now this might sound strange being at either end of your body, but I want you to think about a time in your life when you fancied someone. I mean really fancied someone, so much so that you felt a tingle down below as you passionately kissed them… see the connection! Another great way to relax the jaw is to smile a lot when birthing, particularly after every surge. Smiling creates positive emotions too which can only be a wonderful thing when you are focusing on remaining calm and relaxed.

Always remember: When it comes to applying the hypnobirthing knowledge it must be done correctly to be effective. Your teacher will follow your progress along the way to ensure that you are applying what you have learnt in the best possible way for you.

Hypnobirthing materials

You have either purchased this book online or your hypnobirthing teacher has given it to you as part of your hypnobirthing face-to-face course. This book, in conjunction with the tools and techniques that your hypnobirthing teacher will share with you in class, will ensure that your preparation is complete.

Your hypnobirthing relaxation tracks

Please note: Hypnobirthing MP3s are designed to take you into a deep state of relaxation. You should never listen to any of the MP3s whilst driving, operating machinery or any other activity that requires your full attention.

Your hypnobirthing teacher will instruct you on how to access these powerful recordings. They are a fundamental part of any hypnobirthing programme. Their primary function is to teach you how to relax, switch off the world, and remove any fears, anxieties, worries and limiting thoughts that may be holding you back from enjoying this special time in your life.

Hypnobirthing tracks are proven to promote emotional positivity. Positive suggestions are woven through the sessions to inspire confidence for birthing. Listening to your hypnobirthing relaxation tracks regularly helps to provide reassurance and enables you to focus on your baby's birth in a positive way.

If whilst listening to these tracks you are distracted by any outside noises – a dog barking, traffic, the phone ringing – simply say to yourself, 'I will now double my relaxation and go deeper', or, 'I will now go deeper into relaxation,' rather than coming out of this trance-like state. It is likely that you will be faced with some distractions on your birthing day so getting into the habit of saying these words, as well as practising with distractions, can help you remain deeply relaxed.

If there is a particular word on the track that you cannot relate to, don't like the way it is spoken or don't understand any part of, simply substitute the word for another so that it doesn't become a reason that prevents you from going further into relaxation.

How will the hypnobirthing tracks make you feel more positive?

The most important aspect of having success with your hypnobirthing recordings is repeated listening. This is similar to other things in life where repetition, or daily practice, is one of, if not the most, important part of achieving your desired result. The more you listen to an audio recording, the more the message will become part of your daily life and the more positive you will start to feel.

Daily listening is recommended. Choose a time that is right for you and your lifestyle. You may find that before going to bed, upon waking, or lunchtime are great times to listen to your hypnobirthing tracks, but it does need to work into your lifestyle. Another great time is during a mid-morning or mid-afternoon break or immediately after work. There is no better time to wind down and spend some special time connecting both physically and emotionally with your baby.

Something you can do to enhance your relaxation practice even more is to introduce a particular smell as it will help anchor relaxation. I have always found lavender to be a popular choice due to its calming effects.

'I am really sensitive when it comes to scents, I don't even like perfume. Something I do like the smell of though is Vicks VapoRub so every time I listened to my relaxations I would firstly rub a bit on my chest before closing my eyes. I made sure I took my Vicks to the hospital too so that I had a familiar smell with me that I had anchored relaxation to and it worked a treat. Great for the nasal passages too!' Becky, Herts.

Pregnancy can enhance your sense of smell due to those pregnancy hormones. In this case, oestrogen can make every little scent that wafts your way feel like an all-out assault on your nostrils so be mindful of this when choosing your scent. You may have already noticed that some smells that you liked before you were pregnant now bother you, just as those that bothered you seem more pleasant to your sense of smell. We often talk about pregnancy cravings in class. For me it was custard tarts when pregnant with Frankie and apples with Alana, but when I asked these ladies what they craved, never did I expect responses like these:

'I didn't crave any foods during my pregnancy but I did crave smells. I would carry my daughter's plimsolls around with me in my handbag and pull them out for a sniff on the hour every hour. Maybe it reminded me of my childhood. I'm not sure but I do know I loved the feeling I got with every big snort. I know, very weird indeed!' Simone, Cambridge, UK

'I can't stop smelling the wet bathroom towels and I don't know why, it's just so satisfying.' Ferne McCann, Brentwood, UK

'I experienced nausea quite a bit during my pregnancy and I couldn't get enough ice. I would sit and crunch cups of ice all day long.' Adrienne, Horsham, UK

'I would scoop up the dust behind the oven and sniff it. A dirty craving I know but I just loved the smell of it.' Anna, Welwyn, UK

Chapter 18:

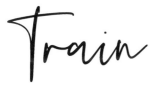

Train yourself to let go

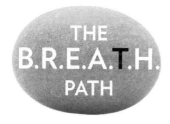

T – Train

In order to become an expert in relaxation you will need to TRAIN yourself to think and breathe the hypnobirthing way. It may feel natural for you to breathe out of your mouth when you exhale but in hypnobirthing you will breathe in and out of your nose except in special circumstances i.e. if your nose is blocked or it feels uncomfortable to do so. It may feel a little strange at first and this is where the training comes in.

'Most hypnobirthing teachers will recommend that you breathe in through your nose and out through your nose. If you can't get comfortable breathing out through your nose then that's fine, simply focus on a slow and controlled out breath through

your mouth. Training yourself to breathe in through your nose and out through your nose prevents gulping for air and, in turn, shallow breathing.

As a general rule of thumb, it is recommended that you breathe in through your nose when practising your surge breathing. This is because when we are anxious we gulp air in through the mouth. As the nasal passages are so small you are unable to do this so there is a natural slowing of the breath. Again, if your nose is blocked or it feels uncomfortable to breathe in through your nose you can of course breathe in through your mouth.'

Tamara x

Words are powerful so train yourself to change a few

Remember, what we think evokes an emotional response and this in turn sets the body up for the appropriate action (perceived or not). You may be so used to certain words that you don't even notice anymore that they are niggling away at your self-esteem. You might want to substitute the following words for another when talking about birth.

PAIN – This word is completely useless in its ability to describe how you are feeling. If one person said they had a sprained ankle, another had a broken one and both were saying they were in pain, how would you gauge how much pain either one was in? The person in pain also has little control over how to change the sensations they are experiencing. It is much better to describe sensations so that you can explore ways of changing them. For example, a tightening sensation can be relaxed, pressure can be eased, etc. The word discomfort is also more useful because we don't compute a negative. To illustrate this, I now want you to NOT think of a white cat. What image do you have in your mind right now? It is a white cat isn't it? Because the brain doesn't understand the negative word discomfort, it has to first explore what the word comfort means and that is much more emotionally acceptable.

CONTRACTION – Even if you choose to change this word to something a little less mechanical sounding like surge or wave, you cannot expect others to do the same. This word has been around for a long time and it is likely that your midwife will use it. I also don't believe it is useful to think of shortening and tightening when you will want to imagine relaxing and opening. I therefore prefer to use the word 'SURGE'.

TRY – As Yoda from Star Wars says, 'Do or do not. There is no try.' When we 'try' to do something, there is always the implication that we may not succeed, which lends itself to the possibility that we may fail. This makes us feel bad, but the reality is that actually we can only do something or not, it is not possible simply to try.

SHOULD – Removing the word 'should' from your vocabulary will take time, patience, and practice. But it is possible to train yourself to do it. Replacing 'should' with more helpful words will lead to a kinder relationship with yourself. Why not replace 'I should start looking for a hypnobirthing course' with 'I could/I want to start looking for a hypnobirthing course'.

NEED – When you need to do something it makes you feel pressured. I want you to feel good about practising so you 'WANT' to do it instead. If you find that you don't want to practise, tap into your conscious desire for change.

Always remember: Hypnobirthing teaches you the importance of routine and practice. It's just like all things in life, if you are not prepared to practice and train yourself until you become good at it, then you cannot expect the outcome that you are wanting to achieve. You need to train your brain to think differently and your body to work in harmony with your thoughts.

Chapter 19:

Hormones

Understand hormones and you will understand birth

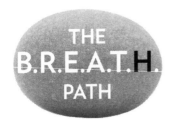

H – Hormones

HORMONES are the 'H' in the B.R.E.A.T.H. Path and they make up the vital ingredients for success. Your hypnobirthing breathing will stimulate the love hormone OXYTOCIN, which is made in your brain and responsible for bringing on your surges. This hormone is also produced when you fall in love and make love, which is why we hypnobirthing teachers call it the very important 'Love Hormone'.

Another very important hormone involved in the birth process are ENDORPHINS. These can help you cope with surges and bond with your baby before and after birth. Focused deep breaths will naturally bring your heart rate more in sync with your breath. This leads your brain to release endorphins, which are chemicals that have a natural calming effect. Without knowing how these important hormones affect your breathing, you might begin to shallow breathe which can inhibit the release of these powerful hormones, making labour much more difficult to manage.

The birthing hormones

Your endorphin levels are also able to rise when they are fully stimulated from the onset of labour, and if their level is maintained throughout, they can actually help prevent your nerve cells from releasing pain signals. But as we have now seen, if there is adrenaline present, this interferes with that balance and severe pain and complications can occur.

Oxytocin, Endorphins, Adrenaline

Through the techniques that you will learn and the support of your hypnobirthing teacher, you will discover how to let go of the negative emotions from the past and reassure your subconscious mind that fearful thoughts have been eliminated.

The techniques will also be teaching you how to become an expert in relaxation, which enhances the ability of the body's natural pain relief, your endorphins. It all consciously makes sense doesn't it? Put like this, it even sounds easy, but most probably you are not totally convinced yet that you can have a comfortable birth experience.

More about oxytocin

It's the love hormone! It produces surges, provides a natural euphoria, helps in birthing the placenta, enables bonding with the baby, and is responsible for milk ejection reflex. Studies have shown that a rise in oxytocin levels can relieve pain – everything from headaches and cramps to overall body aches.

More about endorphins

They are our 'feel good' hormones! Our body's natural pain relief, stimulated by a gentle touch massage. Endorphins are increased by laughter and love, and promoted by oxytocin.

You will learn soft massage techniques designed to stimulate your endorphins, providing a wonderful accompaniment to your hypnobirthing techniques. Your hypnobirthing teacher will guide you through some simple options but it is really up to you both to explore just how you will enjoy this experience. An added benefit to this is that your mind will be distracted away from the part of your body that is experiencing the surge, as you can't help but give your attention to the soothing touch of your partners hands and the enjoyable sensation that it can give you.

Have you ever felt the sensation of a wire head massager? It gives you that goose bump or tingling sensation. It is this feeling that helps to release endorphins in the body. Remember, endorphins are your body's natural pain relief or your 'feel good' hormones. Your partner's gentle and light massage will help you tap into that endorphin system which will help you labour more comfortably. Could you imagine someone cracking an imaginary egg on your head with the yolk running down giving you a chilling sensation? It is this feeling that triggers the hormones you will want more of when birthing.

Your baby loves endorphins too

Whilst bonding, you can nurture your baby into a relaxed and loved little person. Whenever your birth partner massages you, they are soothing and connecting with your baby too. Your baby can pick up on your feelings so when you feel loved and supported by your partner, so does your baby and he or she will benefit from all the wonderful endorphins too. These special hormones will help prepare you for the birth process and motherhood. A ten-minute massage by your partner alongside practising your other hypnobirthing techniques, not only relaxes you but sends a wave of fresh nourishing oxygen to the womb and placenta. It's an intimate opportunity to snuggle up together and pass on thoughts of love and safety to your baby, so establish a practice routine and make every day of your pregnancy as happy, stress-free and precious as possible.

I have often found that babies can become more active when you relax and flood your body with endorphins. It is simply their way of communicating with you by showing you that they too love the feeling they get when you're deeply relaxed. If this occurs, enjoy the feeling of your baby saying, 'Yes Mum, I love this feeling too so make sure we practice lots!'

Adrenaline

This hormone increases your heart rate and breathing rate. Adrenaline triggers the body's fight, flight, freeze or faint response. The body's ability to feel pain also decreases as a result of adrenaline, which is why you can continue running from or fighting danger even when injured. While it can slow down labour if released in the early stages, adrenaline is required towards the end of birthing as it is responsible for the expulsive reflex action of the muscles that help to move your baby down the birth path. I like to think that this is nature's way of helping to make the birthing phase more manageable.

Hormone levels can validate the presence of pain and affect the feelings associated with birthing… it's NOW time to explore PAIN.

Some women experience pain whilst birthing and some don't

I said it right at the beginning of this book and I will say it again. Not I, nor any other hypnobirthing teacher, can promise you that by attending hypnobirthing classes you will be guaranteed a pain-free birth. Saying that, I have proven it can be done and so have many others; but why, if it is possible to have a pain-free birth, can I not promise it?

Expectancy!

This is another example of hypnosis. When we expect that a certain outcome will occur, that is what tends to happen. Sadly, because most women haven't escaped the horror stories over the years, that's what they expect. Whilst they may learn on one of our courses that birth can be more comfortable, they may never completely let go of the belief that it can't happen without pain. The shift from excruciating pain to 'it doesn't have to hurt' is a step too far for some, and can in itself create a fear of not being able to achieve that. I would love for you to experience birth without pain BUT (and it is an important BUT) it doesn't have to be pain-free to be a positive experience. As you progress through your hypnobirthing course, you will learn many things about how your mind and body interpret and affect the sensations you experience.

For some, that leads to labouring in complete comfort and for others they learn how to distance themselves from the more intense sensations. For most, they report back a positive experience no matter what path their birthing takes, one in which they remained calm, relaxed and in control. And whilst we are on the subject of pain let's have a look at it more closely.

Your body doesn't feel pain!

Yes, that's right. Your body doesn't feel pain, or any sensations for that matter. Anything we feel in the body is actually experienced in the brain and the brain chooses what it believes is most important at any given time to pay attention to. If you were to touch any part of your body now you would feel it. I know you know this but give it a go; with your fingers, touch another part of your body. In this moment you are giving your complete attention to that part of your body and so you are feeling your touch.

There are, of course, nerve endings all over your body to ensure that this happens. So, in theory, you should be noticing all of the time, let's say, how your shoe feels on your foot. But you weren't, were you? Not until I suggested you give your foot your attention. We've all heard stories of athletes injuring themselves during an important activity but not noticing until the game is over. I bet when they lose they notice the injury quicker than if they win, too. In this instance, the brain believes the game is more important than dealing with the injury.

Of course it is important to experience sensations in the body otherwise we wouldn't be able to do anything. Let's assume that the sportsman above is a rugby player; without the ability to feel he wouldn't be able to get out on the pitch, let alone run around and catch and kick the ball. Without the ability to feel, we wouldn't be able to experience pleasure; and as importantly of course, we'd have no idea if there was something wrong with a part of our body.

The level of pain we experience is strongly affected by what is most important to us at the time. Back to the rugby player. Maybe instead of getting injured during an important match that rugby player was just having a friendly kick around with his friends. There isn't the same drive to get up and carry on so he's more likely to notice the injury immediately. Pain, therefore, is useful as a tool of communication to let you know when something is wrong at the appropriate time.

How we experience pain is also very subjective. If we were able to administer the same level of pain to two people we may find that one might give the area a rub saying it was unpleasant whilst the other is writhing around in agony.

Both the importance we give to the experience and our emotional state will play a part in what we feel. Think about times when you have been in pain and how that pain varied throughout the day based on whether you were feeling refreshed, happy, enjoying yourself and engaged in something interesting or were feeling tired, angry, tense, anxious or bored. The emotions you are experiencing will impact on the levels of endorphins (the body's natural opiates) being released in order to dampen sensations of pain.

What we are doing will determine the amount of attention we are giving to that part of the body, dictating how much we are noticing the feelings in any given moment. Often pregnant women experience heartburn, backache or other uncomfortable sensations (some quite severe). Some will really have difficulty with these things and others will seem to be able to let go of them quite easily. This could be about pain threshold but it is almost certainly more about how the mind is responding to what is happening and this is the same during labour and birth. Some say that the pain is useful, that it must be there to inform the woman that things are happening and how she needs to respond during labour. I agree you need to feel something, but why does that something have to be excruciating pain? It certainly doesn't appear that way when we watch animals in their natural habitat birth their babies.

'According to physiological law, all natural functions of the body are achieved without peril or pain. Birth is a natural, normal physiological function for normal, healthy women and their healthy babies. It can, therefore, be inferred that healthy women, carrying healthy babies, can safely birth without peril or pain.' Dr John H. Dye, extract from 'Easier Childbirth', 1891

'I have dislocated my knees skiing in the past and that was painful, childbirth was not painful' – Mel, Hertford, UK

'During my first birth the pain was beyond anything anyone could have ever told me. I considered myself to be a survivor of torture. My second birth I did hypnobirthing, I thought about every contraction as bringing my baby closer to me instead of tensing up. I didn't push, I breathed my baby out and I felt like I could have done it all again a week

later. I passionately believe it was my fear that stopped my first baby from coming out'.
Nadia Sawalha, UK Television personality.

How do you view pain?

Over the years I have taught a lot of pregnant couples and I have identified three types of women when it comes to perception or attitude towards pain because, of course, pain is subjective… meaning that what you experience and feel may be very different to what someone else might experience and feel.

Are you a 'pain blocker'?

If you are what I like to call a 'Pain blocker', you absolutely believe that labour will be painful… too painful for you to cope with and you are therefore planning on using pain relief such as an epidural when labour starts. Your primary objective is to not feel any pain at all. You are adamant that this is what you want and nothing or nobody can change your mind. You are wanting to take control of the pain before it takes contol of you. Does this sound like you? You are determined to do whatever you can to make sure that any pain is contained right from the start. You want to block the pain completely by locking it away and plan to take as many pain-relieving drugs as you can get your hands on.

Are you a 'pain waiter'?

If you're what I like to call a 'pain waiter' then you're pretty laid back about everything. You're thinking what will be will be and you're happy to just wait and see what happens on the day and then deal with it then without really thinking about it too much. You prefer to just go with the flow and you'll decide what to do on the day. You might have pain relief or you might not. You're just content to wait and see what happens on the day. Whatever you decide, you're not that concerned by it, because whatever happens simply feels like it is meant to be.

Are you a 'pain embracer'?

Now if you are what I like to call the 'pain embracer', you plan to totally embrace the feelings associated with labour and you're looking forward to experiencing the feelings in labour as a necessary function to meet your baby. You've done all that you can to prepare and educate yourself beforehand and you have equipped yourself with plenty of knowledge and tools to help you manage your labour on the day. You've practised your hypnobirthing and you and your birth partner are focused on the birth that you want. You are feeling ready, prepared and fully equipped to deal with anything that crosses your path on the day. The 'pain embracer' says… bring it on!

So which one are you?

It could be that you're a combination of more than one. I would say I was definitely a 'pain waiter' throughout my first pregnancy because of my lack of knowledge… I really didn't feel prepared at all and I had no idea what to expect. I only attended the free NHS classes that very much focused on all the things that could go wrong. I remember dreading the birth of my baby after those classes.

In my second pregnancy I started off as the 'pain blocker'. I had even planned a Caesarean birth because of the trauma I experienced the first time around. Finding the right education and hypnobirthing enabled me to shift from the 'pain blocker' to the 'pain embracer'. The hypnobirthing knowledge completely transformed my thinking so that I felt fully prepared and I knew exactly what to expect and do when my surges started.

A very small percentage of women will experience a painless childbirth and those that do, well, many keep it to themselves so as not to boast or upset women who say they had a horrible experience. Just because a woman experiences pain during childbirth doesn't mean she hasn't had the right birth on the day.

Always remember: Understanding pain and why some women experience more pain than others whilst birthing is important. Hypnobirthing will never promise a pain-free birth but what it will do is make the feelings associated with birthing much more comfortable, but only after you learn how to remove your fears and have completed a hypnobirthing course. Hypnobirthing helps create the right amount of birthing hormones within your body. It is vital that you understand the importance of these hormones and how they can affect the way you birth your baby on the day.

Path 4

The B.A.B.Y. Path

The B.A.B.Y. Path

A mother's instinct is a powerful force of nature

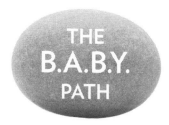

BIRTH PLANNING the hypnobirthing way is the first part of the B.A.B.Y. Path. It is important to know what the **ALTERNATIVES** are when making decisions whilst birthing. Knowing what to pack in your **BIRTHING BAG** can make all the difference to the way you feel on your birthing day. I have included other considerations towards the end of the B.A.B.Y. Path because it is important that you know **Y – WHY** why these considerations matter.

Chapter 20:

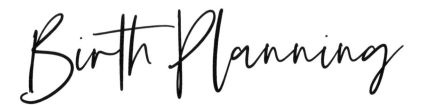

Birth Planning

Your midwife is not a mind reader; create your birth plan!

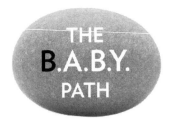

THE
B.A.B.Y.
PATH

B – Birth planning

The 'B' in B.A.B.Y. Path is all about BIRTH PLANNING. Some call this a birth plan and others call it birth preferences (as it sounds more flexible). I believe that it is important to spend time thinking about what you want for the birth of your baby. Spending time beforehand considering what is important will help you make sure that you have what you want both on a practical and emotional level. It will also help you make the right choices for you and your baby on the day should you need to deviate from those plans. Midwives and doctors are not mind readers so you will want to write the salient points down for them.

Keep this short so that they do not feel overwhelmed by the amount of information you are sharing with them on the day, an A4 sheet is about the right amount. Remember that your birth partner will be your advocate during birth so you don't need to put full details on your birth plan. As a birth doula I have always considered myself a walking birth plan. I establish a relationship with the couples whose birth I attend and we speak at length about what is important to them. My role is to ensure that their birth plan is adhered to as closely as possible, which often means reminding other caregivers what a couple's birth preferences are.

By spending time discussing what is important with your birth partner, you will help them understand your expectations of them and they will be more able to support you as you wish on the day. Your hypnobirthing teacher will guide you towards creating a birth plan that is just right for you.

This will enable you to identify any questions that you may have for your midwife or other medical professional, subjects you wish to research further, considerations for your birth environment and how you wish your birth partner and other attendees at your birth to support you. Please remember that birth planning is about what is important for you and this session should not be seen as a checklist of things that you must do, but a guide to the things you may wish to consider.

Choosing where to have your baby

This is an important decision to make as it will not only dictate the environment in which you will birth but also the type of care in terms of who will be present whilst birthing. Here are the options currently available in the UK:

- Home birth.

- Midwife-led unit (MLU).

- Birthing centre.

- Obstetric consultant-led unit (CLU).

Home birth

If your medical and pregnancy history is uncomplicated, then a home birth may be right for you. There is no evidence to suggest that for women with 'low risk' pregnancies, planned home birth is any more or less safe than a hospital birth.

Home births are attended by community midwives, whom you may have already met during your pregnancy. Some women believe that they will be more able to feel relaxed and in control in their own home. If you would like to consider a home birth as an option, you will need to discuss this with your community midwife as soon as possible, so that appropriate arrangements can be made.

Midwife-led unit (MLU)

If you have an uncomplicated medical and pregnancy history, you may wish to opt for midwife-led care. Research shows that if you choose this type of care you are less likely to have your labour accelerated (using a drip with a drug called Syntocinon to speed up labour). You are more likely to be active during labour if you feel like it and get into positions that feel right for you. Evidence shows that women who choose this option are more satisfied with the care they receive, with more consistent advice and greater continuity of care.

After the birth of your baby you will be cared for on the MLU until you and your baby are discharged home to the care of your community midwife. The MLU is often run alongside the obstetrician consultant-led unit, so that if you or your baby experience special circumstances during labour, birth or immediately following the birth, transfer to the consultant-led unit can be arranged quickly.

Birthing centre

A birth centre is normally a small maternity unit that is staffed and, in most cases, run by midwives. They offer a homely rather than a clinical environment. They are good at supporting women who want a birth with no or few medical interventions. Birth centres tend to follow the same rules about care during labour and birth as hospital maternity units.

Obstetric consultant-led unit (CLU)

Obstetric consultant-led care is available to all women. However, those women who have special circumstances are normally advised to birth in the CLU. Pain relief such as epidurals can be accessed here. Midwives continue to provide the main support during labour and birth with input from the obstetric consultant.

Can you change your mind?

You can change your mind at any time during your pregnancy, even during labour. If you have booked into a birth centre, you can decide to stay at home, or if you have booked a home birth you can decide to go to hospital. Ultimately the best environment for you to give birth to your baby is one where you feel safe, comfortable, well supported and relaxed.

Remember, this is a personal choice and what may feel safe for one woman may not for another. There is no right or wrong with your decision of where to birth. If, due to special circumstances, you need to change from your original choice to a CLU, it is useful to recognise that we are incredibly lucky to have the support of skilled medical professionals when nature needs a helping hand. This is key to ensuring that you maintain your emotional control.

Choosing who will be with you when you have your baby

It is likely that you would have never met the midwife who will be attending on the day if you are birthing in the hospital. If you have a home birth planned, then you may find that you know the community midwife who attends as you may have already met her at your antenatal appointments.

Most hospitals will recommend no more than two birth partners attend your birth. However, if you have three like I did, my mum, my husband and my doula, then you may need to pull out your persuasive techniques on the day and always remember this is your baby, your body and your birth. The choice is yours!

A doula

Doulas support women and their families during pregnancy, childbirth and early parenthood. This support is practical and emotional but non-medical in nature. You may find that your hypnobirthing teacher is a doula too.

Independent midwife

Independent midwives are fully qualified midwives who are registered with the Nursing and Midwifery Council (NMC). They have chosen to work outside the NHS in a self-employed capacity to provide pregnancy, birth and postnatal care. I have always found that independent midwives support hypnobirthing and many also have the skills to teach it.

Free-birthing

This is a term used for birthing without any health professionals present. This way of birth means not having any midwifery support, clinical monitoring, or modern technologies during labour. Only a very small minority of women actively choose to birth this way.

Birthing in the water

Getting into water will increase your endorphins and bring about a sense of wellbeing and happiness.

Think back to the last time you had a relaxing bath. Remember as you stepped into the perfect temperature of the water and laid back into the bubbles with a sense of 'ahhhhh that feels sooo good'. For many women getting into the birthing pool can have this same invigorating effect. Remember too that getting into the pool can be the perfect change of environment to promote further relaxation and the feeling of being safe in your own space. If your birth partner is going to join you in the hospital pool you may want to remember to pack their swim trunks; I am sure your midwife will appreciate it.

Your hypnobirthing teacher will show you some beautiful water births in class and share with you why babies won't take a breath until they have come down the birth path and emerged out of the water. I have always found this to be the number one fear when couples are considering birthing in the water. It can be reassuring to know that it can be quite normal for a baby's head to be out in the water for some time before the body comes.

You might also be relieved to know that your baby will not take a breath while underwater. This is because babies are born with a dive reflex which causes them to swallow any liquid rather than inhale it. Exiting the birth path is not what triggers a baby to breathe. Your body is a comfortable 37 degrees celsius and generally the air is not 37 degrees.

It is the change in temperature that stimulates a baby to take a first breath. During your water birth your healthcare provider will frequently check the water temperature. Keeping the water as close to body temperature as possible can help ensure a safe transition so that the baby is not triggered to take a breath.

What if the pool isn't available on the day?

This would of course never happen at a home birth but if all the pools are in use when you arrive at the hospital, you do have the option of getting into the bath instead (only if they have baths). I have always found that midwives are very good at ensuring that once the pool room does become available you will be able to swap rooms. For those parents hypnobirthing on a consultant-led unit you may find that a pool is available to use there also.

Birthing in the water is popular due to the many benefits associated with it

Here is a list of the benefits to you and your baby:

• It is a natural way to help stimulate your endorphins (your natural pain relief).

- It reduces stress and anxiety and, in turn, promotes relaxation.

- The buoyancy of the water supports your weight making it easier to move positions.

- It reduces the risk of requiring perineal repair (the temperature of the water can increase blood flow to the perineum).

- It increases oxytocin (the love hormone).

- It is calming and peaceful.

- As well as providing a safe and private environment, your baby is born into a similar environment to that which it has come from so that they can acclimatise and transition to their new surroundings more gradually.

- It may reduce blood pressure due to the calming effects of being submerged in water.

- Increased satisfaction by allowing you to feel more in control.

Some women prefer to labour in the water for the benefits that are listed above and will then get out of the water when it's time to birth, which is, of course, their personal choice.

Tens machine – another way to stimulate endorphins

A Tens machine (which you cannot use in the water by the way) for labour consists of a hand-held controller connected by two sets of fine leads to four sticky pads that are placed on your back. The machine gives out little pulses of electrical energy that reach your skin via the leads and pads. The pulses may give you a tingling or buzzing sensation, depending on the setting. It is an easy to use, portable and non-invasive machine that can help stimulate your endorphins.

Most women, however, either love it or loathe it at the time and you won't really know until you start to use it on the day as to whether you feel it is helpful for you or not. I have heard many women say that it served as a distraction to get them through each surge and of course this can be combined with your hypnobirthing breathing at the same time. Your hypnobirthing teacher will teach you special techniques serving as a natural alternative to increase those powerful endorphins in your body.

Gas and air

This is a mixture of oxygen and nitrous oxide gas. Some women find that it makes them feel nauseous, light headed, sleepy and unable to concentrate and so quickly stop using it. Other women may describe it as taking the edge off the intense feelings. It is worth mentioning that, as gas and air is available in any location that you choose to birth, a midwife may feel that it is part of her role to offer it to you.

Whilst you may want to use it, a midwife offering it to you may cause you to become more intensely aware of the sensations you are experiencing. Remember that whilst in trance your mind becomes less aware of your body and you feel distanced from it. A midwife asking if you need some gas and air to 'take the edge off' will draw your attention directly back into your body. You may like to include in your birth plan that you do not want your midwife to offer you gas and air and that you will request it should you want to use it.

Other pain relief options

Many women who choose to attend a hypnobirthing course find that they have already made the decision to avoid pain-relieving drugs if they can. Because of this, hypnobirthing does not dwell on the different drugs on offer or indeed their impact on either the mother or her baby. However, should you wish to know more please ask your midwife for more details on this. As with the gas and air, we would recommend that you state on your birth plan that if at any time you want pain relief, you will ask for it. The two most common pharmacological options available are pethidine and an epidural.

Can drugs slow down labour?

If you decide to have an epidural then it may slow down your second stage of labour. It also means that, without the ability to feel as well, your midwife or the monitor you are strapped to will inform you when your surges are coming. It is more likely that an assisted delivery (forceps or ventouse) may be needed to assist in the birthing process. Sometimes less anaesthetic is given towards the end of this stage so that you will be able to feel the sensations and therefore know where to direct your breath appropriately.

Your estimated due date (EDD)

Intervention can occur even before labour has begun and much of this is to do with your estimated due date, also known as your EDD. It is important to emphasise in your mind the word 'estimated'. Firstly, because it isn't about one particular date; there is a window in which most babies are born and that is between 37–42 weeks, which is actually a five-week window. The Royal College of Midwives will confirm this to be true so feel free to quote them with your health professionals if need be.

Secondly, it can take up to four days for the egg to meet the sperm and for implantation to take place, therefore we can't even be sure exactly when the window is. Four days may not sound like a lot of time but it can make a huge difference when looking to avoid intervention. Thirdly, in the same way babies are different sizes and grow at different rates after they are born, so it is when they are growing in the womb.

Therefore, scans cannot be 100% accurate when assessing how many weeks pregnant you are. This is really important if you are sure when conception took place and yet growth scans have caused your EDD to be changed. Understanding this is not only important to help you avoid unnecessary medical intervention but also to help keep you positive should your EDD come and go and your baby has not yet made their appearance. Research shows that less than 5% of babies actually arrive on their EDD so, if you haven't gone into labour before then, it is likely that this day will pass as a normal day.

Hugs before drugs with a large pinch of patience!

Natural nudges to encourage your baby to come

Ideally you will go into labour naturally when your baby is ready to be born. For most, this is between 37 and 42 weeks which is important for you to remember as your excitement grows and perhaps your patience begins to wane.

There are many things you can do to encourage labour to start naturally but the most effective is to utilise what nature has generously provided for us, something I lovingly call 'hugs before drugs'. When we make love, we produce oxytocin. You will remember that it is the presence of the hormone oxytocin, in sufficient quantities, that will ensure that our surges are effective. It is useful to know that both nipple and clitoral stimulation will also produce an increase in oxytocin. The other useful part of making love is that there are prostaglandins in the semen which can help to soften the cervix.

Coming back to the foundation upon which hypnobirthing is based, it will also be useful to ensure that you are not holding on to any fear (be it about birth or anything else), and that you are doing what you can to relax. Of course you will have lots of these skills after you have attended a hypnobirthing course, but another one of my favourites is laughter because of the happy hormones that are produced when this occurs.

'I was 8 days overdue and had tried everything to try and bring my baby on when a friend suggested watching a funny movie. I was half way through the movie when I stood up quickly, laughing so ferociously that gush....my waters released all over the carpet. Ooops!' Jane, London

Other things to consider are to remain active and perhaps seek out the benefits of other complementary therapies, for example:

Reflexology, Acupuncture, Aromatherapy, Hypnosis

Your excited friends and family

Be aware that your family and friends can also bring pressure at this time as they too are looking forward to the birth of your baby. Ask them not to keep phoning and texting and that of course you will advise them as soon as you have your wonderful news to share. If you regularly use social media then coming off or reducing the time spent here will help reduce any unwanted attention from friends and family. When sharing the details of your EDD with friends and family you may want to simply say that your baby is due sometime in that month rather than the actual date.

Considerations during labour

Every woman has different expectations and concerns about what is important to her during labour. We are all different and what may be acceptable to one labouring woman may be completely unacceptable to another. You are, of course, learning many ways to help keep you calm and relaxed throughout labour, even if things are not exactly as you would like them to be, but by planning ahead you are more likely to get what you want. The types of things you may want to consider when planning for your baby's birth may include, but are not limited to, the following:

• How many people would you like in your room?

• Would you like to move freely around the room and get into positions that are right for you?

- Do you have any pain-relief requests?

- Are you happy to have vaginal examinations? Remember this is your choice.

- Who will communicate with the midwife and discuss your birth preferences?

Considerations when birthing your baby

Again this is not a checklist of things that you must do, merely a guide to help you explore options and ensure that you are planning for a birth that is right for you and your baby. The types of things couples consider when planning for their baby's birth may include, but are not limited to, the following:

- Are you happy to use your hypnobirthing techniques rather than any forced pushing?

- Are you happy for your birth partner to gather any information necessary for them to fully understand any interventions suggested?

- Who will receive your baby?

- Who will announce the sex of your baby?

VBAC (Vaginal Birth After Caesarean)

Maybe you have chosen hypnobirthing because of the many benefits it offers VBAC mothers who have already had a previous Caesarean birth.

When we focus on the breath as the baby makes their way down the birth path, it can help with control and thus reduce any stress to the body during this time. If there are any fears relating to a previous birth experience then these techniques can help you feel more positive as you focus on what you want to achieve.

'Watching the VBAC videos on the video library gave me so much confidence to know that if these women could do it, so could I.' Sue, Basildon.

Considerations after your baby has been born

There can be quite a lot of controversy around some of the points given below, with a vast range of differing opinions as to what is the right course of action to take.

Your hypnobirthing teacher will not provide you with their opinion or give advice on what you should do. However, they will provide you with plenty of information in class about the following topics so that you and your partner can decide what is important to you:

- You will learn the benefits of skin-to-skin contact.

- You will learn about birthing the placenta.

- You will learn about the benefits of not clamping or cutting the cord straight away.

- You will learn how to establish breastfeeding more easily.

- You will learn about vitamin K and how is it given.

- You will learn all about the 'Golden hour' and the importance of not rushing this precious time.

Birth planning together is a must!

Your birth plan is a written record of what you would like to happen during your labour and after your baby is born. You may have heard people saying to you 'it all goes out the window on the day so don't worry about a birth plan'.

If there is nothing in writing then your caregivers will simply follow protocol and the chance of receiving the birth you want will be greatly reduced. It is important to be flexible and have an open mind. Your hypnobirthing techniques will help you deal with any change of plans along the way.

Reflecting back to what you learnt earlier, unless you know that intervention is likely due to an existing special circumstance, hypnobirthing does not recommend that you focus your attention too much on medical interventions.

However, some couples feel that it is useful to have this information to help, should they need to deviate away from their ideal birth. This is why I have included a short description of the main forms of intervention in the next section.

Always remember: Don't even think about not writing down your birth preferences for your caregivers. They are not mindreaders and they need to know what is and what isn't important to you. Your hypnobirthing teacher will provide you with plenty of information to support your individual birth preferences and encourage you to explore different options using reliable sources.

Chapter 21:

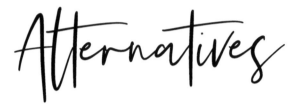

It is important to know what the alternatives are when making your decisions

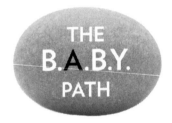

A – Alternatives

Induction of labour

In my experience of supporting pregnant women and their partners, it is clear to see that way too many couples have felt the pressures of looming induction. It seems as if it is quite normal for many midwives to start talking about induction just as soon as a mother has reached her estimated due date.

I was induced for no medical reason at 11 days past my EDD with Frankie, and then with Alana I was determined to let nature run its course. I went 13 days over my EDD with no interference, meaning I simply carry babies longer than other women and that's what is right for me.

I am not anti-induction, there certainly are times when it is needed, but the induction rate is currently at an all-time high so please be aware of this and ask lots of questions if you find yourself in this situation. Your hypnobirthing teacher will be a great person to support you so that you can make the decisions that are right for you and your baby.

Induction of labour is a process designed to start your labour artificially. Induction is generally carried out when the risks of continuing pregnancy outweigh the benefits. It is usually more intense than spontaneous labour and epidural analgesia, making the need for pain relief and an assisted delivery (using instruments such as forceps or ventouse) more likely to be needed.

If you choose to be induced, ask your midwife or doctor to discuss the induction process with you fully. The choice is always yours, so make sure you fully understand the medical reasons in order to make an informed decision. I urge you to find out what the induction rate is in your area and ask what the reasons are as to why it might be so high, before deciding to take the induction path.

A membrane sweep

An optional membrane sweep is often offered as a routine procedure to women who have passed their EDD (estimated due date). Your midwife will carry out this procedure. During this internal examination, she will sweep a finger around your cervix (neck of your womb) to separate the membranes from the amniotic sac surrounding your baby from your cervix.

This separation releases hormones (prostaglandins) that could start labour. If you have had a baby before, then a sweep may be offered to you at your 41-week appointment. Remember it is always your choice and you can decline it. Your hypnobirthing teacher will share with you many great alternatives that can gently help nudge baby along.

Why would you be offered an induction of labour?

Induction of labour is offered for a variety of reasons where it is felt that giving birth sooner would benefit the health of you or your baby. This may be because of special circumstances such as:

- Diabetes.

- Pre-eclampsia.

- Concern about baby's health (growth and development).

- Size of baby.

- Previous history issues.

- Mothers who have received IVF treatment.

- It is often advised that twin/multiple births are induced.

- If you are an older mother then induction may be advised.

- Scans, however not always accurate, can determine a baby's size.

- Stillbirth.

'When is it better to induce labour than to let a woman's body or baby decide the best time for birth? What are the pros and cons of waiting and of being induced? What about after the due date? When the baby is thought to be bigger than average? When the woman is older? If she had IVF? Or when her waters have broken earlier than usual? Induction of labour is an increasingly common recommendation and more and more women find themselves having to decide whether to let their body and baby go into labour spontaneously or agree to medical intervention. This book explains the process of induction of labour and shares information from research studies, debates and women's, midwives' and doctors' experiences to help women and families become more informed and make the decision that is right for them.' Extract from 'Inducing Labour: Making Informed Decisions' by Sara Wickham[5]

5 Wickham, Sara; *Inducing Labour: Making Informed Decisions*; Birthmoon Creations; 30 April 2018 (2nd edition)

Medical interventions for birth

An instrumental delivery (ventouse/forceps delivery)

If there is a special circumstance and your midwife or doctor feels that assistance is required to help get your baby out, then birthing instruments may be offered to you. The instrument that's best suited to your particular circumstances will be used. Both forceps and ventouse (vacuum or suction cup) instruments have different risks and benefits, which your doctor or midwife will take into account when discussing your options with you.

What is an episiotomy?

An episiotomy is an incision that is made to the perineum area to assist the birth of a baby. Anaesthetic is used to numb the area beforehand if this is required. Please ensure that you understand and accept the reasons given to you as to why this procedure has been advised and remember your decision-making process that your hypnobirthing teacher will guide you through. If you do decide to have this procedure whilst birthing then your hypnobirthing techniques will be most valuable.

The Caesarean birth rate is rising

In 2018, the UK Caesarean rate was just over 26%. This is slightly higher than the previous years. In countries like the USA, Spain, South America and Australia it is much higher. It has been reported that the Caesarean birth rate in Brazil ranges around the 80% plus mark in their private hospitals, and over 50% in their public hospitals.

Elective Caesarean birth

A Caesarean birth is an operation where your baby is born through an incision made through your tummy, most commonly across your tummy just above your bikini line, but occasionally a vertical (up and down) incision may be used.

If a special circumstance is identified that means the benefits of an elective Caesarean birth outweigh the risks for you and your baby, the reasons will be explained to you.

Booking an elective CS after my traumatic birth felt like the best option, my only option, the safest option and by doing so it gave me the control back. It wasn't until I met a doula named Suzanne who completely changed my way of thinking. I cancelled my CS the day before I was due to have it because of the niggling voice in my head saying....but what if this hypnobirthing stuff really works, surely I must give it a chance

Tamara x

If your plans change and a Caesarean birth is required can you still have a hypnobirth?

Those women who have special circumstances and are advised to have an elective Caesarean birth will still very much benefit from the hypnobirthing education. The hypnobirthing knowledge is beneficial and transferable to any sort of birth that you have. Your teacher will show you how to adapt what you have learnt for any type of birth.

Knowing about hypnobirthing will help you to:

- Let go of any anxiety surrounding the Caesarean birth using the knowledge, skills and techniques learned in class.

- Use your tools to remain calm, relaxed.

- Understanding the birth process and know your options.

- The relaxation practice can have a calming effect on your baby. Should you wish, your hypnobirthing teacher will be available for additional support with regards to adapting what you have learned if your plans need to change along the way.

Emergency Caesarean birth

I spoke about curve balls earlier and yes sometimes even couples that have covered all bases with their birth preparation cannot foresee some special circumstances that may need an emergency Caesarean birth. There can be many reasons for this such as a baby showing signs of distress, problems with the placenta or umbilical cord, position of baby or labour not progressing. The reasons for this decision will be explained to you and you will be asked to sign a consent form for the operation. Should this occur, your hypnobirthing techniques still remain important for helping both you and your birthing partner to remain calm, relaxed and in control.

Breech is another form of normal, some may say

Sometimes the only reason you may require a Caesarean birth is because your baby is in a breech position with their bottom or even feet presenting for birth rather than their head. Unfortunately, within the NHS, it is usually considered too high risk to go ahead with a natural birth. Although there are some NHS midwives available to deliver breech babies, many lack the confidence that is required.

However, hypnosis can be a very effective tool to turn a baby that is in a breech position and therefore, before accepting the inevitability of a Caesarean birth, you may wish to have a breech-turn hypnosis session as soon as you realise that baby is in this position. You can ask your hypnobirthing teacher if this is something they can offer, otherwise they may know someone that they can recommend.

'Emma was 40 weeks plus three days pregnant when her midwife discovered that her baby was breech. She had planned to birth at home and I had even dropped off my pool in a box for her to practise with the week before. The fairy lights were up, affirmations covered her walls and, as her doula, I was on call and ready to leave as soon as she needed me.

So what did Emma do?

- *She asked for a scan to confirm baby's position.*

- *Went onto the Spinning Babies website for more information: www.spinningbabies.com*

- *She made an appointment with the consultant to talk about her options and these were the questions she asked:*

  — *"How successful is an ECV (manual turn of the baby)?"*

  — *"If I birth my breech baby vaginally in the hospital will there be qualified staff here to do this?"*

  — *"How likely will it be that these staff members will be on duty when I need them to be?"*

  — *"What is the closest hospital with the highest breech birth rate available?"*

  — *"I don't want my legs in stirrups when birthing… What are the options?"*

  — *"Can I birth my breech baby in the water on the MLU?"*

  — *"Can you provide me with some statistical research to back up your views?"*

Emma decided an ECV was what she wanted to do and I sent her a breech-turn hypnobirthing script to listen to also. It was music to my ears when I received the following text the next day, "I listened to the track at the same time as having the ECV which wasn't really that uncomfortable at all and it worked! My baby is now head down, just being monitored so fingers crossed she likes it this way up and we are back on for my home birth."'

Tamara x

What is an ECV?

External cephalic version (ECV) is a process by which a breech baby can sometimes be turned from presenting bottom down or foot/feet first to head down. It is a manual procedure that is recommended by national guidelines for breech presentation of a pregnancy with a single baby, in order to turn the baby for a vaginal delivery.

What exercises can help?

The hip tilt

Lie on the floor in front of a sofa or chair, with your feet on the sofa or chair. Place a pillow/cushion under your hips for additional support. Your hips should be elevated above your head, and your body should be at a 45-degree angle, a bit like a mini shoulder stand in yoga. Hold this position for 10 to 15 minutes, three times a day. It's best to do this when your baby is active. Listening to a hypnobirthing breech-turn-script recording can also help. That way you are working with both the body and mind at the same time.

Sit on your birthing ball and rotate your hips

Sit on your birthing ball and once you have found your balance, gently rotate your hips clockwise in a circular or spiral movement. Repeat 10 rotations and then change direction, rotating your hips counter-clockwise for 10 rotations. Repeat this three times a day. Closing your eyes and imagining your baby in the optimum position for birth can also help.

Rocking your baby

Place your hands and knees on the floor so that you have created a hammock-like position for your baby. Keep your hands and knees in place as you gently rock your body back and forth for as long as feels comfortable to you. Repeat up to three times a day, and you may wish to put a pillow under your knees for this one.

Stay active – walking and swimming

Walk, do pregnancy yoga with a specifically trained prenatal teacher who can ensure you and your baby are safe and looked after, swim, or engage in another low-impact exercise. Do this for 30 minutes a day. Staying active may help your baby move out of the breech position.

All the above exercises can be done whilst listening to your hypnobirthing tracks to help keep you relaxed and focused mentally on what you want to achieve.

'I tried absolutely everything, and I mean everything, to turn my baby. From ECVs to hypnosis to Moxibustion, I researched and met with consultants, asked for second opinions, changed hospitals and in the end I made the informed decision to birth my breech baby vaginally. It was amazing and apart from having a lot of people in the room with me that day I just kept my eyes closed, focused on my hypnobirthing breathing and totally believed in myself and my baby. I actually think birthing my breech baby was easier than birthing my first.' Georgia, Bishop's Stortford

Protocols

There are many protocols within the maternity care system. They are there to standardise the care that you are given so that you can receive the best evidence-based care available. What this can do is pigeonhole you as belonging to the same group as all other birthing women. And what I mean by that is, when something happens that does not fall within the guidelines or protocols of the place you have chosen to birth in, then intervention is often suggested. Yes there is a lot of contrasting practice out there and I see it a lot, particularly when I attend home births or births on the MLU (midwife-led unit) as opposed to the CLU (consultant-led unit).

I have always noticed that midwives have a lot more autonomy at home births and on MLUs which is probably because they are being left alone by the hierarchy of the hospital setting and the obstetricians. Just for the record, I have met some truly incredible obstetricians in my time and we are lucky to have them when nature needs a helping hand, so just to clarify I am not anti-obstetrician. However, you may find yourself in a situation where you will need to question or even ask for a second opinion before you make any decisions about yourself and your baby. As a doula I work alongside the midwife and we support each other to ensure that the birthing couple receives the best possible care, and it is wonderful when I witness consultants being respectful of the birthing woman's domain; however, I have also been in plenty of situations where this hasn't been the case.

I think using the word guideline instead of protocol makes it sound more flexible and it should be, because all women and all births are different and they should never be pigeonholed. Flexible guidelines... now that sounds much better! This reminds me of a conversation I once had with a midwife colleague who was questioning the way they practsced where she was working.

'The senior midwife warned me that she would grab the emerging baby if I didn't follow hospital protocol and do a "hands on" delivery rather than watch the birth with my hands poised. I'd personally risk a lot to do the best for the woman in my care but at times I've decided that means staying quiet and doing what I am told so as to not disturb the woman's faith in us health professionals. This doesn't always feel right.' Anonymous

They said I wasn't allowed so I can't

I am constantly around pregnant women and I have lost count of the amount of times I have heard the words CAN'T and ALLOWED. You are not at school now and I am sure you fit into the category of being a responsible adult so why do so many women say that their midwife or doctor said that they weren't allowed to have a water birth, they can't birth at home, they are only allowed to have one birth partner in the room, they can't get into certain positions and, the real biggie, they are not allowed to leave the hospital? If anyone does any allowing it is you!

Now I am not saying you need to do the opposite to what the medical professionals are advising, I am just explaining what they are doing. They are advising or recommending or sometimes even strongly recommending, and that's fine. You are always allowed and you always can when it comes to your body, birth and your baby so please know that this is your starting point before you make your birth choices.

You do have the human and legal right to make decisions that are right for you and your baby. This also means that you should not have any options denied to you during and after you have had your baby. I have always found that hypnobirthing gives women and their partners the strength to stand up for themselves and question what might be going on so that they can weigh everything up and make informed decisions together.

Hypnobirthing can help you bring control back if you find yourself going off track. When you also have a supportive birth partner who is on the same page as you and will speak up as your advocate if required, then you will find that you will be able to better deal with any situations that could arise on the day. One of the most powerful things about hypnobirthing is that it helps you cope with whatever turn your birthing takes on the day.

'There is a wider issue of compliance to those in "white coats" that can affect all of us and is not purely a woman's issue. Most of us, male and female, have been conditioned to accept without question that "doctor knows best" and to follow their "orders". However, there is something about being female that makes challenging authority of any kind particularly difficult, perhaps because, as young girls, looking around us as we grow, most "authority" is male.' Give birth like a feminist, Milli Hill[6]

The fear release hypnobirthing script

Quite simply, if you don't remove your fears around birthing, trying to create a positive expectancy of birth will be like building a house on wet sand. Any positivity will be in constant conflict with the negativity that is stored within the subconscious mind.

6 Hill, Milli; *Give Birth Like A Feminist*; Harper Collins Publishers Ltd; 2019 (1st edition), page 37

Your hypnobirthing teacher will take you through a fear-release hypnosis session in class. It will enable you to release any emotional issues, fears and concerns that you have, clearing your mind of all potential negativity, to enable you to focus on your labour and birth in a more positive, confident way.

Unfortunately though, there are plenty of opportunities for others to share negativities with you that could affect your confidence. However, the hypnosis session is only a part of the process, as you will also want to consider any other issues that may cause upset as you approach your baby's birth. Some examples of this follow.

Practical preparations for the new arrival

- Is your home ready for your new arrival?

- If you are undertaking any major building works and they won't be complete, what needs to be finished?

Coping as a new mum

- How are you feeling about becoming a mum? This is as equally important if this isn't your first child as the dynamics of your role will be changing.

- In particular, think about those first few months and what kind of support you will be expecting from others. This is the time to communicate those needs, rather than worry if it will actually be available to you.

- If there isn't that support from close family, look at what strengths you must build to effectively provide your own best support.

- Spend time talking with your partner about the type of parents you each want to be and how you want to bring up your child. Are you on the same page?

- Think about how bringing a new baby into your life can affect your relationship.

- Do you have any concerns about the impact having a baby will have on your career?

- Do you have any conflicts with needing to work and wanting to stay at home with your baby?

Sorting through these types of questions can help you reconcile with what you really feel you want to do. No matter what your list reveals, spend time discussing the practicalities of resolving any issues and look for ways to make your peace with those that you cannot.

Always remember: There is nothing more important than knowing what all your options are. There is always an alternative for you to consider when it comes to birthing your baby. Hypnobirthing will open your eyes to many aspects of the birthing world and ensure that you become better informed around the subjects that are specific to the birth you want to achieve.

Chapter 22:

Birthing Bag

Knowing what to pack in your birthing bag can make all the difference to the way you feel on your birthing day

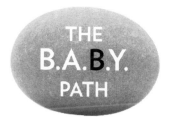

B – Birthing bag

It is important to take some supplies with you on the day in your BIRTHING BAG particularly if you get hungry. As a hypnobirthing mum who understands how fear affects the body during the birthing process, it is likely that, because you have plenty of oxygenated blood in your uterus muscle, your digestive system which is also located in this part of your body will be functioning normally too. Therefore, the feeling of hunger can be experienced. Yes, you can eat whilst birthing if you feel like it.

As a doula and as a part of my hypnobirthing classes, I like to share the contents of my birthing bag. I'm not saying you need to go out and purchase everything on the list but it will give you something to think about.

Possible contents of a birthing bag

- Hypnobirthing tracks and relaxation music. Remember your phone charger!

- Scents: If you have anchored relaxation to a particular smell throughout your hypnobirthing practice then take that with you.

- Food: Think high-energy foods that require little preparation and not a lot of chewing. Fruit purees are high in sugar and quick and easy to consume. Pasta is a slow burning carbohydrate and therefore great to eat in the early stages of labour.

- Drinks: If you like coconut water, pack it. Otherwise think high-energy drinks and plenty of water. Camomile tea is always good to offer everyone in the room particularly if anyone needs calming down.

- Lip balm, eye mask, ear plugs, ear phones, phone, flannel (can be made warm or cold), heat pack, socks, sanitary pads, massage oil, battery candles, images, affirmations, birthing ball.

Items to pack for your baby

Nappies, Clothes, Hat, Car seat, Blanket, Cotton wool, Water wipes.

> Always remember: Once your hypnobirthing bag is packed you will feel more ready and organised knowing that you have everything you need to enhance your comfort on the day.

Chapter 23:

Y - Why

It is important that you know Y (Why) you will need to consider these suggestions

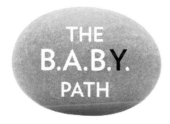

Y – Why

Without knowing WHY, you can't make an informed decision. The following considerations might be useful to you and your baby. You may miss out on the benefits of them if you don't consider them. You may not resonate with everything in this next section, but knowledge is power and I want you to be as informed as you can possibly be. In this section I have included a brief explanation of WHY you may want to consider these topics as part of your antenatal preparation and choices.

WHY delayed cord clamping?

This is a huge subject to cover and deserves much more attention than I could ever include in this book so I urge you to do some further research on this topic. The benefits of delayed cord clamping are hugely related to the health and wellbeing of your baby. Your hypnobirthing teacher will cover how, when and why you need to consider this important option for your baby.

WHY is knowing about the placenta important?

The birth of your placenta is known as the third stage of labour. Most women discard the placenta straight after the birth of their baby but others keep it. You will soon read why below.

WHY use an umbilical cord tie?

Your baby has an umbilical cord that connects from their abdomen to the placenta, which in turn is connected to your uterus. More and more couples are choosing cord ties once the umbilical cord has been detached because not only are they pleasing to the eye but softer on your baby's skin. Umbilical clips are made of a hard plastic which can dig into a baby's tummy if caught under their nappy.

WHY some couples choose a lotus birth

Again this book is not long enough to cater for this subject, so please do some further research if this interests you or even ask your hypnobirthing teacher about it. A lotus birth simply means leaving the placenta and cord intact until it comes away on its own after a few days. The placenta is carried around in a special bowl or bag with the baby, until it drops off.

WHY using a birthing ball, birthing stool, the cub or peanut ball can help

It is all about getting as comfortable as you can be on the surface that you are resting on. They help with positioning and opening your pelvis in order to help your baby come down the birth path. You may find that your hypnobirthing teacher will show you how to use these wonderful birth tools in class. You may find they are available in some hospitals too, but if not you can of course take your own.

WHY more women are packing the 'rebozo'

Every birth I have ever attended I have used my rebozo. It is a very strong Mexican scarf that can be used to help unborn babies move into better positions, a wrap for comfort and massage. A rebozo scarf can even be used to hold onto and provide support when getting into different birthing positions e.g. squatting.

WHY aromatherapy is used whilst birthing

Aromatherapy essential oils from plants can be used to enhance physical and mental wellbeing. The oils can be massaged into the skin, dropped into a bath or a few drops placed into a steam diffuser. It is a great way to help you relax even more and I have found that many more midwives and doulas are training so that they can offer the benefits of this. Always make sure you have sourced a qualified aromatherapist when using these oils for pregnancy and birth.

WHY a 'blessing way' or a 'baby shower' is arranged

Many couples choose to celebrate this special time in their lives. How lovely it is to empower a new mother for her journey of birthing and motherhood. It is a time to welcome the power and strength that is already intrinsic in women's bodies, and to shower her with love and support. Whatever they choose to call their celebration it is an acknowledgement of this special time in their lives and that they will soon be bringing another life into the world.

WHY some couples keep the sex of their baby a secret

Who really knows why some people find out and others don't? We are all different and we all value different things. What's tricky though is when only one of you wants to know and the other doesn't. This can make for some interesting conversations in order to persuade the other to agree to it or not. I would say it is pretty much 50/50 when it comes to finding out the baby's sex. Only half prefer to have the surprise and the others are not too bothered by the surprise element. 'Gender-reveal' parties are becoming increasingly popular as a way of bringing friends and family together to celebrate this momentous occasion.

'If I had found out the sex of my baby during my 20-week scan it means I would have had 20 weeks of listening to what those around me thought about what it means to have a boy or girl. I think part of the motivation to keep going in labour was the surprise at the end of it all'. Sally, Bedfordshire

In the absence of a conclusive sex scan I have always found it interesting the way people attempt to determine whether a baby is male or female. Some say if you're 'carrying high' it's a girl, and low means it's a boy. If you're craving certain foods; sweet, they automatically say girl while sour equals boy. Someone may even swing a pendulum across your tummy to confirm the sex for you. But guess what? 50% of the time they guess right, every time!

WHY some women choose to keep souvenirs of birth

Okay, when I say souvenirs, I mean parts of the baby that are left behind and often discarded immediately after birth. What I am talking about is keeping the placenta, the membrane and the umbilical cord. Now I totally understand that this is about personal choice, but unless I make you aware of what some women do you won't really know whether you would like to do it too.

Let's take the placenta – you can keep it all intact (see lotus birth). You can encapsulate it, drink it and eat it. There are proven health benefits associated with keeping the placenta and let's face it, animals eat it after they have birthed their young because of how rich it is in iron and hormones.

'I remember my doula asking if she could take away the placenta with her. I said "if you want it you can have it" as I had no real desire to do anything with it. There

was something really sacred though when she returned it to me having baked it, ground it up and put it in a lovely jar. She said I could use it for medicinal purposes and I did once when I applied it to Alana's bottom when she had nappy rash, and guess what? Her rash was completely gone the next day.'

Tamara x

Now you might be thinking why keep the cord and the membrane? If you were to gently wash them and put them into a shape, a love heart or even the word 'love' and waited a week or so for them to completely dry you may be pleasantly surprised by what you have created.

I have also seen images where placentas have been placed onto a piece of paper to create a keepsake, and the uncanny likeness to a tree imprint is pretty incredible.

If you do decide that you would like to do any of the above, please add it to your birth plan so that your midwife knows, and remember to pack a suitable air-tight container with you.

WHY knowing about different positions can help

An inspirational mentor of mine and founder of the Active Birth movement, Janet Balaskas, says there are two words to remember when it comes to birth positions and they are 'upright' and 'forward'. Every birth that I have ever witnessed where a mother was in this position, where gravity was assisting, has always birthed far more easily than any mother lying down. You will have lots of fun with your birth partner when you practise birth positions in your hypnobirthing course.

WHY change positions and when?

Whenever you feel like it, is the right answer. If your midwife has examined you and it appears that you are fully dilated (10cm) or you get the urge to bear down with a downward pressure in your back passage, then it's time to get into the birthing position of your choice and focus on your bearing-down breath. If you find, however, that your baby is not coming and you have been breathing this way for 20 minutes then you may wish to consider a change of position. Sometimes just a change in position is all you need for your baby to turn and make their way out.

When hypnobirthing meets Active Birth

Throughout my career as a hypnobirthing teacher I worked alongside the wonderful Janet Balaskas at the Active Birth Centre in London. It is here that I launched The Wise Hippo Birthing Programme® in 2013. Myself and Janet would spend hours chatting about positioning and female physiology. Janet is the founder of Active Birth and a world-recognised name within the childbirth community. We made a great team and together we would attend midwife events calling our talk 'When Active Birth meets Hypnobirthing'.

Janet describes hypnobirthing as the education that perfectly complements active birthing. It's a meeting of the body and mind. When the two come together, working perfectly in sync like the two sides of a beating heart, birth preparation couldn't be more complete.

'In an "Active Birth" the mother herself is in control of her body. She moves and changes position freely – she is the birth giver. Whereas in an actively managed birth, all the power is taken from her, her body is controlled and she is a passive patient. An Active Birth is one where the first resort is the mother's own instinctual and natural resources and the last resort is medical intervention.' Janet Balaskas, Founder of Active Birth

Ligaments and pelvis

I have already shared with you why you and your baby are designed the way that you are when you explored the B.O.D.Y. Path; however I wanted to add a little more. Learning how your body works at the end of pregnancy and during childbirth is very helpful as you prepare for birth. When you understand what is happening, you can interpret your body's signals more effectively and participate more fully in your labour and birth. The pelvis is made up of two large bones joined by cartilage and ligaments at two joints in the woman's lower back, at the sacrum (called the sacroiliac joints) and at the front symphysis pubis bone. During late pregnancy, hormones soften and relax these ligaments making the pelvis elastic rather than rigid. This gives the pelvic bones the ability to stretch and open more easily for the birth of the baby. Your pelvis is not fused and stretches and opens for the amazing process of birth. Being upright and forward lets gravity help the pelvis to open and aids the descent of the baby during labour.

The physiology of the baby's head

It is also worth mentioning again that as your baby is making their way down the birth path and getting ready to be born, the bones in the skull overlap and reduce in circumference. This means your baby's head will reduce in size at the moment of birth, making it easier for your baby's head to come out. This is exciting don't you think? You and your baby, both working together. Nature giving you both a real helping hand! You'll notice two soft areas at the top of your baby's head where the skull bones haven't yet grown together. These spots, called fontanels, allow a baby's head to move down the birth path by transforming into a cone-like shape. Your baby is so very clever!

WHY you need to know what to do if labour slows down

Sometimes labour can start and then stall, weaken or even stop. This can be normal and, as long as there are no special circumstances, you may find that you will just want to wait and be patient. If you are birthing in a hospital then the time that you arrive will be noted and if for example your waters have released, the medical staff will want to see that your labour is progressing within a particular time frame. Here are some suggestions that you can use to bring labour back on if you feel the need to get things moving again:

- Have a nap and listen to your hypnobirthing tracks.

- Have a warm bath.

- Go and sit on the toilet: the feeling of releasing and letting go is helpful.

- If you feel like being active then it can help to walk up stairs sideways.

- Sitting on a birthing ball.

- Eating something to provide energy.

- Think about increasing the oxytocin as it is the oxytocin that brings on surges.

- Nipple and clitoral stimulation.

- Soothing strokes to increase endorphins and oxytocin.

- Watching something funny. This will help promote relaxation and in turn increase the oxytocin. The downward thrust of the breath caused by laughing is also useful.

- Whilst relaxing, imagine baby moving down.

How to speak with medical professionals

It is incredibly important to prepare for this in advance due to the effect of 'shock' hypnosis I mentioned earlier in the B.R.A.I.N. Path. Remember, if you are hearing new and difficult information without preparation, this will side-track the conscious analytical part of your brain. When this happens we naturally follow whoever has the most authority.

Whilst this may well be the appropriate course of action, too many couples share that they wished they had trusted their instincts as they believe that they were taken down a path that didn't feel right. It can be daunting though for some to question what they are being told by a medical professional and the following can help keep you focused.

Remember to take your 'BRA' with you!

What are the BENEFITS of following the course of action suggested? What are the RISKS involved? In particular ask what the immediate dangers and specific medical indications are (i.e. something that is actually happening not something that might happen). Ask about the ALTERNATIVES (and the benefits and risks of these). Follow your instincts. This is important because it doesn't matter what anyone else would do in your situation, it is about what feels right for you personally. Whilst birth partners will be more than likely asking the questions and will have most probably come to a decision themselves, the final decision must always be that of the mum. Only she can tap into what is actually happening within her body and with her baby.

Ask what would happen if you did nothing. Buying time, even if it is for only 15 minutes, can make the difference between intervention or not. Everyone is on the same team and that means working to ensure mum and her baby are healthy. Asking questions isn't about being antagonistic, but about getting professionals to think outside the box and not treat all women the same. By asking questions, and making decisions based on the answers you are given, you will maintain control of your baby's birth. As mentioned previously, even if the decision is to hand your birthing over to the medical team, you will have maintained your control by ensuring that it is the right decision for you and your baby.

If you do accept intervention at any point ensure that, should this lead on to the suggestion of more intervention, you use your BRA again. If conversations around intervention are required prior to labour starting, I would strongly recommend that women take their partner with them to any appointments. . Take your BRA with you, be informed, and make the right decisions for you and your baby.

benefits, risks, alternatives

Why knowing the signs is important

All women in labour are different and there really is no set pattern. If you have had a baby before, then it is also likely that this labour and birth will be different. You will use the techniques in a way that is right for you. Labour can start in a number of ways. If this is your first baby then I am sure you are wondering how you will know whether your labour has started or not. Here is a list of signs, in no particular order, that can indicate labour has started or is getting ready to start:

- Surges have started (often intermittent to begin with).

- Membranes have released (maybe the water is trickling out slowly, or maybe it was more of a gush).

- The uterine seal has come away (a sign that your cervix is thinning).

- Tightening sensations in abdomen, lower back or thighs.

- Vomiting or loose bowel actions.

As soon as you discover that your labour has started it is important to remain calm and relaxed throughout, and by now you will have learnt and understood all the reasons why this is so vital. The best thing to do is to just carry on as you are, be patient and let labour progress slowly. Even if you do not feel you need to, as each surge comes in close your eyes and do your hypnobirthing breathing. This will ensure that you are stimulating your endorphins right from the outset and setting the scene for how you wish to be as your labour progresses. If labour does start progressing quickly, then have your partner time your surges so that you can gauge when it is time to phone your midwife. There are plenty of mobile phone apps out there to help you time the surges more effectively.

If labour starts during the night

- Sleep for as long as you can.

- If you can't get back to sleep, put on your hypnobirthing tracks and stay relaxing in bed or somewhere else of your choosing.

- This is a time when you would normally be sleeping, so if it is the early stages of labour aim to stay resting if you can.

- Remember to remain calm and not get too excited. I would recommend not waking your partner unless you really need to as they will need their energy to support you when the time comes.

If labour starts during the day

- Continue with any activity that is comfortable for you. It is important to listen to your body and rest if you need to.

- If you are resting, find a position in which you can be most comfortable. Set the intention 'to be as comfortable as you can be on the surface you are resting on'.

- Relax through your surges with your hypnobirthing techniques.

- Follow your body's lead, breathing as deeply as you need to.

- Listen to your hypnobirthing tracks, or any music that you find relaxing.

- Watch or read something light-hearted and funny. Laughter relaxes the pelvic area and helps to focus on the downward motion within your body.

- You may want to have a bath, go for a walk and eat something to keep your energy up.

- Enjoy this early indication that your baby is going to be with you soon.

- When to call the midwife: Check with your own midwife what the procedures are in your area as they can differ. Make sure you have the correct phone number written clearly at the top of your notes so that you and your partner can easily find it when you need it.

If I am having my baby in a midwife-led unit or hospital, when do I go?

- Listen to your body and trust your instincts.

- If you have a long journey to the hospital (distance or length due to time of day), you will want to leave earlier than if you live very close by.

- Find a balance between enjoying relaxing in your own home and ensuring that you will be able to remain calm and relaxed on the journey. I know it's exciting but you must remain calm as excitement can produce unwanted hormones within your body (adrenaline).

- Take your time when walking to and from the car. As a surge comes in, put your arms around your birth partner and breathe with your hypnobirthing breathing. There is no need to rush. Stop, pause, lean forward, breathe and relax until the surge passes before going any further.

Practical considerations for hospital births

- Check in advance how long it takes you to get there during busy and quiet times.

- Find out if there are different entrances that are dependent on time of day.

- Find out what the car parking arrangements are and how the pay machine works.

- Think about where you will feel more comfortable sitting or lying down in your car.

- If possible, your birth partner requests a midwife skilled in hypnobirthing.

- Your birth partner should discuss your birth preferences and expectations with the midwife (ensure they do this again if there is a shift change).

- You will settle down and listen to one of your favourite hypnobirthing tracks or music.

- If you have been active at home prior to setting off, you may find that you want to rest on arrival. Listen to your body and trust your birthing instincts. Do what feels right for you.

Other practical considerations

- Bring extra copies of your written birth preferences in case of a shift change.

- Take your own pillow with you.

- Dim the lights in the room if you can (newspaper and tape can be most effective at blocking out the light).

- Bring snacks and drinks.

To push or not to push with the 'bearing down breath'?

I like to call this particular breath the 'bearing down breath' for two main reasons:

- If you feel the need to roar like a bear during this time to birth your baby then that is exactly the right thing to do. Just because you may have been fairly quiet up to this point as you focused on breathing through your surges and listening to your hypnobirthing tracks, it doesn't mean you need to stay quiet now. This is such a primal moment.

- The second reason is because I have heard many birthing women describe what it feels like as exactly this… a bearing down sensation rather than a pushing sensation.

When it is time for your baby to make their way down the birth path, there is no need to do lots of forced pushing. This is a very outdated concept and comes from a time when women used to be anaesthetised and unable to birth their babies, so instruments were used to assist the baby's entry into the world.

Forced pushing is stressful on both mum and baby and can, in fact, slow things down as it closes the sphincters of the vagina ahead of the descending baby. It can be an overwhelmingly exhausting experience for a woman. This is where your cleverly designed body comes into play and it's known as 'the natural expulsive reflex action'. When this occurs it gently helps to nudge your baby down the birth path.

'I felt like my body had gone into automatic pilot mode and I couldn't have even stopped it if I tried. I know my baby was working just as hard as I was and I could feel her coming down like a corkscrew. It was such an incredible sensation; both of us working together to make it happen.' Delphine, London

Unlike other techniques you will learn on your hypnobirthing course, you can't practise birthing your baby, but you can definitely imagine and dream. However, there is another function within the body that uses a similar natural expulsive reflex action. Have you guessed what it is yet? Of course you have, it is when you are opening your bowels. Think about it – you don't think to yourself, 'Do you know, at some point today I'm going to want to poo, so I'll go and sit on the toilet for the next few hours and push with all my might until one comes out.' Of course you don't. You wait till you get the sensation that you need to. This is exactly what you want to do when you are birthing your baby, and because you will be using the same natural expulsive reflex you can practise your 'bearing down breath' whilst opening your bowels on the toilet.

The more you practise the 'bearing down breath' the more you are learning how to tune into the natural expulsive reflex of your body, and experiencing how the 'bearing down breath' and focused attention can enable everything to remain relaxed and open easily. When the time comes to have your baby you will be fully prepared to work with your natural expulsive reflex to help nudge your baby down and out.

Remember that during the birth of your baby you are the expert regarding when and how to bear down. You should not need to be given outside instructions regarding this unless you want it. It is important to just go with the flow of your body and trust that your body and your baby will know what to do. Despite new midwives now being trained that forced pushing is not necessary, it still may be useful to put on your birth plan that you do not want any outside instruction from anyone when you are birthing your baby. Women who choose to have an epidural are less likely to feel this sensation and are therefore often encouraged to push.

Whilst you focus on your baby moving down you may like to say the word 'OPEN' in your mind. Or you may just like to imagine your baby coming closer to you with each surge. As I said, don't feel that you need to be quiet. Not all women are and a powerful, bear-like, primal, vocal birth can be just as incredible as a quieter birth. If you feel the need to make noise at this time then go with what your body is telling you to do. Sometimes the need to make these primal noises is part of the process of helping you to release and let go.

Remember, if you find that you have been bearing down for a considerable amount of time then you may want to think about a change of position; sometimes a change in position is all you will need so that your baby can turn and come out more easily. Remember those three important words when positioning your body for birth ... upright and forward! If you watch a woman in labour who is more active and upright, you will notice that she may instinctively start to rock her hips or to move her pelvis in a spiralling motion. This can help your baby move down more easily.

As you approach the end of dilation you may start to notice that you need to change how you are breathing. This is the time that you will want to start your 'bearing down breath'.

- Follow your instincts with the 'bearing down breath'.

- If you feel as though you might be losing control, go inward and keep the breath slow and controlled.

- Follow your body's lead.

- Assume whatever birth position feels right and comfortable for you.

Using your imagination with the 'bearing down breath'

As you are bearing down you may like to imagine your baby moving down the birth path by imagining the opening petals of a flower when your breath reaches your pelvic area. Remember it is important to do what feels right for you at this moment. Imagining a flower at this point may help you to focus inwardly giving you more control over the feeling. Your hypnobirthing teacher will guide you through this breath and encourage you to practise daily. This breath will help you feel more in control as your baby is coming down the birth path.

Remember your body and baby will follow your thoughts and feelings. During this time, mums often just like to know their birth partners are there and any suggestions can be spoken quietly and lovingly.

'Go with what your body is telling you it wants to do, trust your instincts, just follow your body's lead. Every surge is bringing you closer, focus on your breath, you can do this.'

Tamara x

If labour starts quickly

Sometimes labour will commence very quickly. This may, in the first instance, cause you to feel out of control. If this happens it is important to remember that you have been practising how to access a calm and relaxed state quickly and easily. You are in charge of your mind and your thoughts and this is of particular importance to understand if the surges arrive quickly and intensely with little or no warning. In the first instance you will want to remind yourself that you know how to take control of your breathing and in turn your ability to cope with the sensations. As a surge begins to come in, you will breathe exactly as you have been practising all along. Between your surges you can imagine that you are resting in your relaxing or favourite place in nature. During your hypnobirthing course you will be guided towards achieving this with ease.

Birth partner's checklist on the day

• Hand over antenatal notes to midwife.

• Discuss birth preferences with midwife/health professionals.

• Ensure the environment is as perfect as it can be.

• Consider how many people are in the birthing room.

• Ensure music/relaxation tracks are on in the background.

• Does mum have a favourite scent to enhance relaxation?

• Give drinks and snacks when necessary.

• Use endorphin-enhancing, light massage techniques.

• Remind mum of facial relaxation.

• Use anchors, suggestions, read scripts.

• Look out for signs of tension and use relaxation techniques to bring her back to a state of calm.

- Whisper positive, loving comments: 'you can do it,' 'I love you so much,' 'you are calm and relaxed.'

- Comfort her and be by her side.

- Hold her hand.

- Gauge her temperature and see if she needs more or less warmth.

- Oxytocin stimulation if needed (nipple and clitoral, loving hugs, massage).

Why skin-to-skin contact is important straight after birth

Once you have birthed your baby they will be placed on your bare chest immediately after birth for skin-to-skin contact. Place a towel/blanket over your baby to keep him/her warm and avoid any bright lights from going in your baby's eyes, so that they can slowly acclimatise to their new surroundings. Some midwives will suggest putting a hat on baby's head immediately after birth whilst others are more relaxed about it.

Skin-to-skin benefits include:

- Regulates baby's temperature.

- Calms and relaxes both mother and baby.

- Regulates heart rate and your baby's breath.

- Stimulates digestion.

- Enables colonisation of baby's skin with mother's friendly bacteria, thus providing protection against infection.

- Stimulates feeding behaviour.

- Enhances the release of hormones to support breastfeeding and bonding.

- Skin-to-skin contact (or 'kangaroo care') helps preterm babies to be more stable, maintain their temperature, fight infection, grow and develop better and be discharged from the hospital sooner.

- Microbiome benefits.

What is the microbiome and why is it great for your baby?

A mother's microbiome (I like to call this her friendly bacteria) and the benefits and research associated with this subject are still being discovered, but it is an area of high interest in the birthing community. More and more women are adding this to their birth plans, even those choosing a Caesarean birth.

'Just before I went in for my Caesarean birth I asked the midwife if the obstetrician could insert a gauze inside me so that they could then wipe it over my baby's face. I had thoroughly researched this topic and it's what I wanted to do. Apparently they don't do that sort of thing at this hospital yet. It must still be early days with acknowledging that this is a thing to do.' Loraine, Welwyn

The birth path is full of necessary bacteria for your baby. Babies receive their first microbiome from their mother when they come down the birth path. During that journey, a baby gets completely covered with bacteria, giving them a brand new microbiome that is necessary to build a strong, healthy immune system. Babies receive this microbiome in three main ways:

- When they come down the birth path.

- Skin-to-skin contact.

- Breastfeeding.

Birthing your placenta

You may need to remind your midwife if you are planning a natural third stage (placenta delivery) and not to clamp or cut the baby's cord until it stops pulsating. If you are planning on taking your placenta home with you, then please ask your midwife to put it into a plastic bag or take a container with you. Some mothers who have chosen to encapsulate their placenta will have a private specialist come and collect it directly from you. It is becoming more common to ingest the placenta afterwards in the form of a smoothie or capsules. This is an area for research if it is something that interests you.

'My placenta wasn't coming out, so my doula suggested I go sit on the toilet and focus on my hypnobirthing breathing again. Sure enough five minutes later it was out.' Cleo, St Albans

WHY breastfeeding is important

A baby's sense of smell is very powerful and they will love the natural smell of you, so when washing yourself after birthing avoid applying soaps, creams, perfumes etc. to your chest area. Your normal and natural smell, even if you are slightly sweaty, is what your baby prefers and this can help establish breastfeeding more easily. Most mothers and health professionals feel that breastfeeding as soon as you can after birth has many benefits. To find out more about breastfeeding please ask your midwife or hypnobirthing teacher where you can attend a breastfeeding education class. There are many breastfeeding support groups around the UK, so ask your midwife where you can attend a support group if you feel that you need a little help in this area.

Some hypnobirthing teachers will incorporate breastfeeding information into their classes or even offer an additional class to specifically focus on this. If not they will know who to recommend in your area. Breastfeeding cafes and support groups are a popular place to meet other breastfeeding mums and gain the support you may be needing. When a pregnant couple logs into The Wise Hippo website they are able to access plenty of videos to support their learning along the way, including an informative breastfeeding class. Mums also receive postnatal MP3s to support their journey into motherhood.

'I wanted to breastfeed my baby so badly but I never knew it could be so tricky, she just wasn't latching on properly. I went to one session at my local breastfeeding support group and the lovely lady, a volunteer I think, sorted it straight away. I am so glad I never waited.' Jo, Cheshire

WHY hypnobirthing is great after the birth, too

Many couples find that using their hypnobirthing skills after their baby has been born has many benefits too. If you happen to get yourself into a situation where you start to feel nervous, apprehensive or even scared, then your learnt breathing can help bring you back down to a state of calm. It's a great tool for life rather than flying off the handle which never helps anyone. Because you would have anchored the feeling of relaxation to your hypnobirthing music you can continue to listen to it whenever you need to take time out for yourself and just relax. Remember your baby may find your music soothing too because they learnt how to relax whilst in your tummy due to all the hypnobirthing practice you will put in.

'As soon as I put the music on, her little eyes rolled back, she stopped crying and a real sense of calm came over her face. Six months on, she goes to sleep listening to her hypnobirthing music every night. This might be the reason why she has slept through the night since she was only seven weeks old'. Susanne, Essex

WHY booking a 'closing the bones' session can help

Now you might be thinking what on earth are you talking about Tamara, and I get it. I agree it sounds a little strange and although I don't really like to use the word trend, this procedure is trending or, if you prefer, growing in popularity. I've had it done a couple of times and I loved it, it made me feel really special. You may find that your hypnobirthing teacher also offers this alongside everything else that she does. So what is it?

Firstly, 'closing the bones' is a ceremony and a celebration of motherhood. It is a postpartum healing ceremony, which was created to nurture the mother after giving birth and embarking on her journey into motherhood. Closing the bones is a tradition from Ecuador, where the postpartum mother is blessed, anointed, massaged and wrapped (a traditional Mexican shawl called a rebozo is often used). The ceremony focuses on closing the hips through nurture and relaxation. This can be done alone with a practitioner, or others close to you can be invited to attend the ritual.

'Having had a traumatic birth I thought this would have conjured up all sorts of repressed emotions but it didn't. It in fact made me realise how much I have now made peace with what happened to me and my baby that day. Even though I was wrapped up like a giant colourful caterpillar there really is something truly incredible about women being there 100% just for you. In my life as a mother of two, I give give give, so for the tables to be turned like this was totally out of my comfort zone but it made me feel almost invincible, like a queen for the day. It's hard to put into words really, you just have to try it for yourself.'

Tamara x

WHY a postnatal (afterthoughts) session can help

Many hospitals now offer something known as an 'afterthoughts' appointment or a reflection session. This is where you can go in and discuss the birth that you had there so that you are not left wondering why certain things happened along the way. If you have been left wondering why things unfolded the way they did then this is a way to find answers to your questions. I do find, however, if a woman and her partner have done hypnobirthing then their birth knowledge is of a particular standard which will complement the conversation in terms of the questions you need answered. You will be able to discuss any memories, your feelings and thoughts during this confidential session. The midwife will talk through your birth notes with you so that you can understand what happened during your birthing. This is particularly useful if you are planning to have another child in the future.

'I attended an afterthoughts session not long after my baby was born and it really helped me put my mind at ease. I never did really know why the midwife was encouraging me to push so much but now I know why and I feel much better about it all.' Fiona, Surrey

WHY self-care as a new mum is vital

You will be so focused on being a mum once your precious baby is in your arms that you may even forget to get dressed or even brush your teeth some days and that's okay. Becoming a mum is a journey and a new path altogether which this book doesn't cover. However, continuing to use your hypnobirthing techniques is a great way to continue to remain calm and relaxed during any challenging times.

A good idea would be to keep in contact with your hypnobirthing teacher too because she will have a wealth of knowledge to signpost you to any postnatal classes throughout this time, whether it be breastfeeding support, mental health support, baby yoga, baby massage, buggy exercise classes, water baby classes, singing and signing classes or new mum meet-ups in your area.

Enjoy this special time with your baby as it sure does fly by, but ensure that you also take time out for yourself, and what I mean by that is finding an activity to take care of your mental, emotional and physical health. Good self-care is key to improved mood and reduced anxiety. It's also key to your happiness with the relationship you have with yourself and those around you. Self-care can simply mean getting out into the fresh air for a stroll around the park, now that is great for both you and baby at the same time!

'I attended my local breastfeeding support group on a Monday, baby group on a Tuesday, Mum would meet me at the pool on a Weds so I could go for a swim (my self-care!!), Thurs was stay home day and Fri is always coffee morning with the other mums I met in my hypnobirthing course... being a mum is exhausting!' Simone, Hertford, Herts.

Always remember: During your hypnobirthing course you will gain much insight into why things are important during the birth process. When you know 'the why' it will help you make the necessary informed decisions that are just right for you and your baby. You will come away from your birth experience with so many reasons why hypnobirthing was a great way for you and your partner to prepare for birth.

Concluding Thoughts

My two birth experiences could not have been more different. I don't like to go into detail about the birth of my first child as it was very traumatic for us all. I was induced for no medical reason the day the Twin Towers went down, so I definitely know how fear can affect a woman in labour.

After that experience I swore I would never ever do it again, until I became pregnant five years later, which came as quite a surprise. The thought of having to give birth again was just too terrifying for me so I booked an elective C-section thinking that was my best option at the time.

I was 36 weeks into my pregnancy when I stumbled across hypnobirthing purely by chance and I feel so lucky that I did. To be honest, I always had that voice in the back of my head saying, 'this sounds too good to be true,' but something was telling me I must give it a go, especially when I read that babies that are born using these techniques experience less trauma, sleep better, feed better and are calm in nature because they have learnt to be this way with all the relaxation practice.

In preparation for my second birth, I trained myself not to be frightened by learning how to get myself into a deep state of relaxation quickly and easily. The affirmations I listened to must have been hugely responsible for the change in my attitude and mindset.

The hypnobirthing knowledge gave me the confidence I needed in my body's own ability to birth naturally. I was determined to outnumber the hospital staff this time so I had my mum fly over from Australia and I hired a doula. This time I went 13 days past my EDD before going into labour naturally at 5am on the first day of spring 2007. Two hours later we phoned the midwife who told me to call an ambulance as my surges at this point were very close together. I had no intention of calling an ambulance and when Serg asked if he could have a quick shower before we left I agreed, really showing how calm and in control I was. I lay on the back seat of the car with my eyes closed and listened to my relaxation music. I think I actually fell asleep at this point as I remember being woken up abruptly by the speed humps upon entering the car park at the hospital.

My midwife said I was unable to get into the water as I had had a previous traumatic birth. Now I know that this was not a good enough reason to deny me the birthing pool. I could see that they were short staffed and I suspect this was the real reason.

My mother transformed my room on the CLU within minutes to a relaxing environment with music, the smell of lavender and pictures which made me immediately feel more comfortable. My position of choice was to lie on my side on the bed where I stayed in a deep state of relaxation for around five hours (it felt like around two hours to me) until I felt the need to get onto my knees and breathe my baby down. I birthed a 9.5 pounder, completely pain free, the feelings were intense but I never ever even considered pain relief, not even gas and air. I loved every moment of it! I could feel her nudging her way down at the same time so I knew she was helping me and we were working together. My daughter was born with the amniotic sac membrane still covering her head which is quite rare and my waters released as her body came out. I remember thinking how clean she was, having been washed on her way out.

I birthed on the bed, on my knees with the top of the bed raised. When the moment came to breathe her out I just focused on the techniques I had practised many times before and she entered the world so gently, without any forced pushing whatsoever. I picked her up and put her on my bare chest straight away and she lifted her head, opened her big blue eyes and just stared at me... What a moment!! She then started to look around the room with a real knowingness before snuggling down and finding my nipple. She latched on within minutes of being born and she instinctively knew exactly what to do.

I had no idea that birthing could be so beautiful. What a contrast to my first birth! My husband was so amazed, he couldn't even tell when I was having a surge because I was just so calm and relaxed as I breathed through each one with ease. My doula on one side and my mum and Serg on the other. I remember feeling safe and so completely focused on staying calm as I birthed my daughter.

It was later that very same day that I began to wonder why it was that all women didn't know about hypnobirthing. It has to be the easiest and most natural way to birth and if I could do it, anyone could! I felt like I had just discovered one of the world's greatest secrets.

'Small steps in the right direction can turn out to be the most empowering steps of your life'

My birth experience was definitely an epiphany in my life, as it immediately set me on the path to becoming a hypnobirthing teacher so that I could share this wisdom with others, and I have never looked back since. If I can be a part of preventing women from having to go through what I did during my first birth then I know I am definitely on the right path. It's the best job in the world and I feel blessed to have found my true purpose in life. Not only was my path changed that day but when my mum flew back to Australia she was greeted by my sister, Rochelle, announcing she was pregnant again. The timing couldn't have been more perfect for my mum to embark on her new career as a hypnobirthing teacher too. It was time to show my sister what she had been missing out on during her previous births.

I couldn't wait to hear her birth story and what words she was going to use to describe her experience this time.

'Jessica's birth was amazing, I felt so in control this time in fact out of all six births I can honestly say I thoroughly enjoyed this one!' Rochelle, Paynesville, Australia.

On reflection, I find it amazing that when you feel things are falling apart in life it can actually mean that they are falling into place. My hypnobirthing experience created a triple transformation within my family and may it continue when all my nieces and nephews have their children in the future. I know Aunty Tamara's book will be the first thing they receive.

Knowledge is power

It is now time to see whether you have experienced a transformational experience in any way. What five words would you use to describe childbirth now?

1 ....

2 ....

3 ....

4 ....

5 ....

Now go back to page 46 and compare the words you originally used to describe birth. Have your words changed? If they are more positive in nature that's fantastic showing you how education can influence your thoughts and feelings. However small or large the differences may be in your descriptive words just imagine how much your confidence levels will improve after you have completed your hypnobirthing course.

For many more inspiring hypnobirthing stories, please visit The Wise Hippo Facebook page at https://www.facebook.com/thewisehippo/ and visit The Wise Hippo website here: www.thewisehippo.com

To find out where you can find a passionate teacher near you please visit www.thewisehippo.com and click on the 'Find a teacher' directory to find a course that is just right for you. Do that and I know you will achieve the right birth on the day for you and your baby!

'Hypnobirthing gives birth to well-educated mothers and supportive birth partners who know how to face their fears head on. Together they learn to trust and connect in both mind and body, creating the harmony that is necessary to make informed decisions that are just right for them. They develop tools for life that can aid them far beyond birthing. If nature needs a helping hand along the way then it's great to know that these tools can transfer to any situation, no matter what path your birthing takes. Now that you have explored all four paths and discovered all the benefits of hypnobirthing there is just one more choice for you to make in order to complete your journey. Finding a great hypnobirthing teacher is now highly recommended to help you kick your fears into touch and is the way to go from this point onwards. I wish you, your partner and your baby a memorable and positive pregnancy and birth experience that on reflection you will describe as having achieved "the right birth on the day"!'*

Tamara x

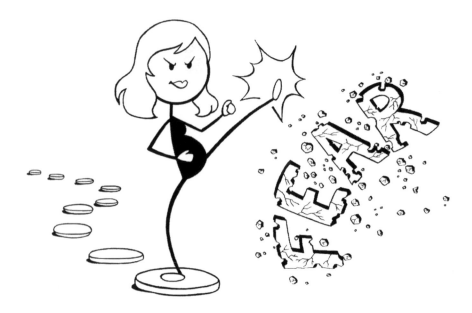

PS…

There's nothing like a last-minute addition to a book and talk about perfect timing!

Only two weeks before going to print a lady by the name of Hilary contacted me with her birth story… Wow, another early report on the use of hypnosis before the phrase 'hypnobirthing' was coined, so, of course, I had to include it!

Below is Hilary's personal account of her birthing. The details of the full report are in the footnote. [7]

OK Relax

'For some time alternative medicine has become increasingly important in pain relief. My experiences of hypnosis in childbirth have convinced me that the use of hypnosis for pain relief generally, should be more widely available.

Labour during the birth of my first child was long, painful, confusing and frightening. Despite having attended classes and read the right books, I found myself wired up to a foetal heart monitor that kept cutting out, needed banging to get going again and was not actually being monitored in any case. I used the gas and air for pain relief, but at one point the cylinder ran out and my husband couldn't find any nursing staff to replace it for some time. Both these factors left me feeling frightened and extremely vulnerable.

Second time round I was determined that I should feel more in control. My husband, a psychologist, was researching hypnosis at the time and I had already acted as his subject many times for experimental purposes. It was when I was using the gas and air, that the effects reminded me how it feels to be hypnotised. I decided that if ever I were having another child, I would give hypnosis a try.

---

7 Graham, Hilary (Moon); 'OK Relax' blog article adapted from *British Journal of Experimental and Clinical Hypnosis* (1984) Vol 1, No.2, pp.49–52 by Hilary and Tim Moon

We duly discussed our ideas with my GP and midwife and both were in agreement. Prior to the birth, my husband and I discussed the type of words or suggestions that might be helpful during labour. We came up with floating, drifting, warm and comfortable and so forth. I was also hypnotised and given a key or trigger word that would immediately enable me to go into a deeper hypnotic trance. In my case we chose 'OK relax'.

On the day of the birth I went into the GP Unit of the local hospital and by 7.30pm the routine paperwork was taken care of and I was settled into the bed. Time to begin.

At the start of the next contraction, my husband gave me the trigger words backed up by the type of suggestions already discussed. Once each contraction was over, I was able to chat normally to my husband and the midwife was able to examine me. This pattern continued until I was ready to push; at this point I felt no further need for hypnosis.

I found the whole experience intensely interesting. Firstly, even during the frequent and strong contractions near the end of the labour, I had coped well with the pain. I knew there was pain, but I felt distanced from it and untroubled by it. During each contraction, I remained in exactly the same position, sitting up in bed with my hands resting on my legs. For some reason this exact position became important. I also sweated quite a lot although I was not apparently moving at all.

The whole event was relaxed and at times comical. On one occasion, my husband had gone to the toilet between contractions. On hearing me call him as the next one was starting, he rushed out and caught himself in his zip. There he was, with the half-hypnotised midwife in hysterics, trying to keep a straight face as he put me into another trance.

Just one hour and 25 minutes after we started the hypnosis, Anna was born, without the use of pethidine or any other drugs. She was immediately alert and looking around the room – no doubt seeing what mischief she could get up to.'

Huge thanks to those who shared their inspiring birth stories with me.

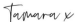

Printed in Poland
by Amazon Fulfillment
Poland Sp. z o.o., Wrocław